The Mindful Eating Method

The Non-Diet Way to Natural and Pleasurable Weight Loss

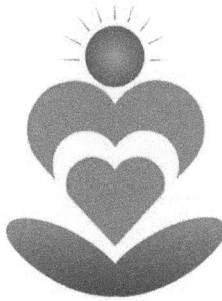

Elizabeth "Lily" Hills

The Mindful Eating Method

The Non-Diet Way to Natural and Pleasurable Weight LossElizabeth "Lily" Hills

2020 Print Edition

www.TheMindfulEatingMethod.com

*****

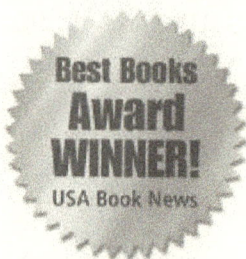

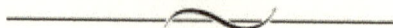

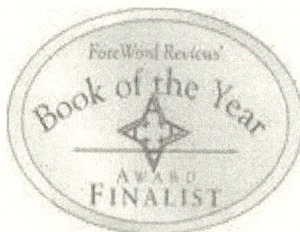

Winner USA Book News National Best Books
Award – Health, Diet and Weight Loss

Finalist Foreword Magazine's Self Help
Book of the Year

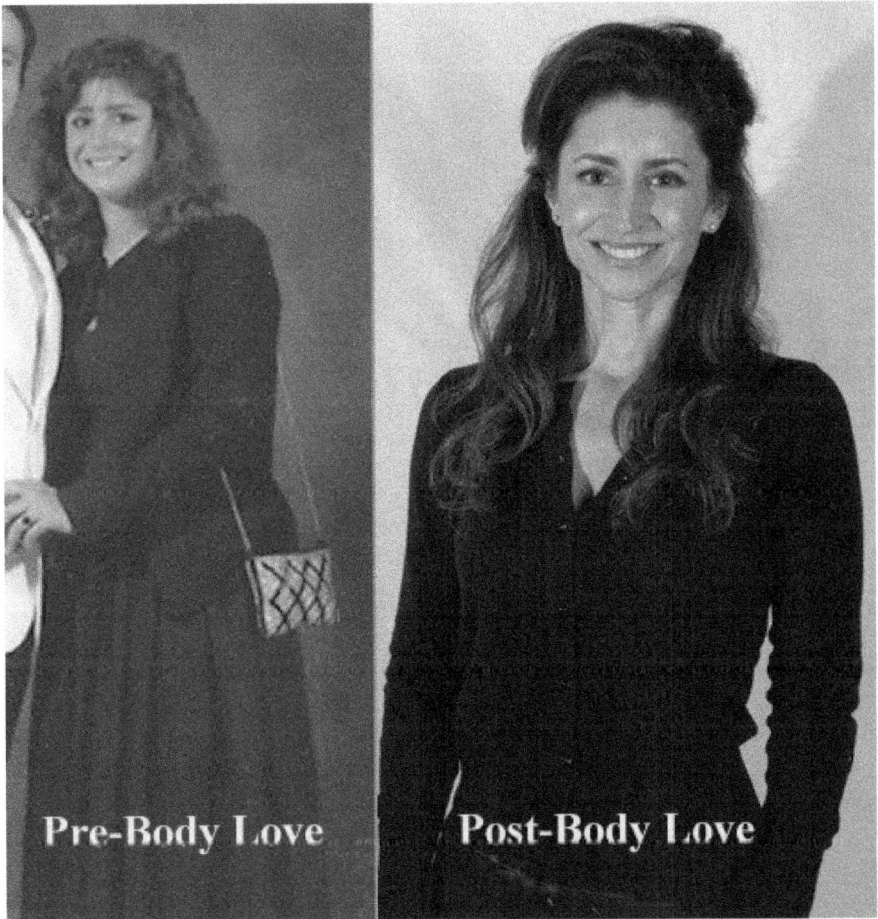

Pre-Body Love   Post-Body Love

What Others are Saying About The Mindful Eating Method...

"A work of monumental importance to modern women everywhere."

Juliette Frette The Examiner

By gently leading you beyond gain and loss to an awareness of you loving essence this book, The Mindful Eating Method, can change your life. I highly recommend it. –

Dr. Leonard Laskow, Author of Healing With Love

"This is the best book I have read on weight loss and body image. Lily knows from which she speaks, and I thought as I read it, "She gets it!" She has discovered a loving way to deal with the issue, which is both simple and transformative. She also speaks to you as your body, to give you a prospective on what you are doing to yourself. We all know "diets don't work", and this is not another diet book."

Kathrine, Amazon Review

"The Mindful Eating Method, singled out by USA Book News in the health category, is filled with concrete suggestions and practices that, if followed even only in part, will help those, as its subtitle suggests, "love the body" they have and "create the body" they want."

Leslie Katz – The San Francisco Examiner

"A must have book for mastering your inner power, and applying your "unlimited potential."

Mindquest Reviews

Note to readers…. Don't forget to check out the additional resources referred to at the end of the book or go to

www.TheMindfulEatingMethod.com

*****

The Mindful Eating Method

The Non-Diet Way to Natural and Pleasurable Weight Loss

By Elizabeth "Lily" Hills

First edition copyright 2011 Elizabeth Hills

Post Office Box 4886

Carmel, CA 93921-4886, U.S.A.

This book is available in print from most online retailers

ISBN 978-09819388-5-1

Disclaimer

This book is intended as a guide to understanding natural and non-compulsive eating, not as a medical manual. It is not intended as a substitute for any treatment that may have been prescribed by your doctor. Consult your medical practitioner before beginning this or any new eating program, especially if you are dealing with an illness of any kind. As I am not a medical professional, or doctor, I am making recommendations based upon a set of lifestyle practices that have allowed me to overcome a compulsive relationship with food and achieve my healthy and natural weight and I am not offering medical care, advice or treatment of any sort.

Table of Contents

*****

Dedication

To all of the loving and beautiful people I have met on my life journey who have helped me to find a loving and gentle voice within myself. I am the woman I am today because you touched my life.

*****

"The single greatest contribution you can make to this world is to know, appreciate, respect and love yourself, exactly as you are today."

–Anonymous

Introduction

Our Story

What Happens When We Don't Love Our Body

Do you ever feel like you can't stop eating, even when you *really* want to? Do you find yourself eating large portions of food that you're really not hungry for and then beating yourself up for your lack of willpower? Have you been trying to lose weight for so many years you've lost count? Is a huge amount of your self-esteem connected to what you weigh? Do you find yourself ashamed of your body, even sometimes resentful of it? Have you been so desperate to conquer your food and body image issues that, short of walking down a crowded street completely naked, you would do just about *anything* else to be rid of the obsession?

I can relate *intimately*. For well over a decade of my life, I had a compulsive relationship with food that dominated my thoughts virtually every waking moment. I was utterly addicted, plagued beyond comprehension by overwhelmingly powerful urges to eat far more than I was truly hungry for. I could hardly go a few moments without thinking food-related thoughts, such as:

"I ate too much."

"When can I eat again?"

"Is this bread allowed on my diet?"

"I'll start my diet tomorrow, and I'll have that pizza now."

Anyone who has experienced it knows that thinking obsessively about food gets old...fast. It is incredibly tiring, stressful and depressing. Additionally, my mind was all too often fixated on a never-ending loop of thoughts that were highly toxic:

"I look terrible."

"I'll never lose weight."

"I have no self-control."

"I hate myself."

"I wish I had a body like that girl."

This obnoxious tape of debilitating thoughts played over and over in my mind, and I felt totally powerless to stop it. My unrelenting focus on the same obsessive, disempowering thoughts took a big chunk of the joy out of every day. While still a happy and fulfilled person in many other ways, I knew my compulsion with food was a giant barrier to my true potential for happiness.

I ate for a *huge* variety of reasons, very few of which were related to being truly physically hungry. My binges were misguided and futile attempts to make myself feel better, to feed emotional hungers for greater levels of love, appreciation, fulfillment, affection, excitement, peace, connection and happiness. I also ate because I was avoiding my uncomfortable feelings, especially worry, frustration, confusion, fear, boredom and insecurity. Food was my sole stress management tool. My compulsive eating was an attempt to shut out the negative and sometimes downright mean "voice" in my head, the one that was making me feel bad by picking on me:

"You didn't get enough done today."

"Your thighs are too big."

"You are not good enough."

Or getting me to worry about something that might or might not happen in the future:

"You're not going to make it on time."

"You'll never get it all done."

"Something might go wrong."

I tried to escape the discomfort created by this negative internal dialogue not just by eating, but also by zoning out in front of the television, or shopping, or cleaning or overworking. When I was alone and I *really* allowed myself to take a good hard look at how I was living my life, without any of my usual distractions, I would get deeply depressed. As I didn't like feeling sad and dejected, I'd quickly return to my default distractions so I could numb myself to my inner turmoil once again.

Having anesthetized myself through food for so long, I became increasingly unwilling to face and feel some of my intense feelings of worry and insecurity. Just as with avoiding paying bills, the longer I delayed dealing with my emotions, the larger the "fees" I paid. At the time, it was much easier for me to sneak an extra snack, or five, to quiet the uneasy feelings that were making me want to escape my body than it was to dig in and deal with them directly. I didn't even know where a lot of these uncomfortable feelings originated. What I did know is that if I denied myself food when I wanted to eat, I felt high anxiety, which is why I didn't often resist eating for long. Like a friend, food provided solace when I was stressed or fearful, entertainment when I was bored, and a welcome distraction when I was overwhelmed or confused.

In addition to my extensive laundry list of excuses to binge, I also ate because I was depressed over having gained so much excess weight. Although admittedly eating did give me a *temporary* break from my uncomfortable feelings, the distressingly tight clothing that was a consequence of all those binges gave me another reason to feel bad about myself—and another reason to eat. So I ate more and more, until I couldn't take another bite, until my stomach protruded painfully, and I'd swear to myself for the umpteenth time that this was my *very last binge. It* was the classic, ugly vicious cycle.

My weight fluctuated erratically for twelve years. I felt ashamed of my body because it looked so disproportionate to me, so different than I wanted it to look, so unlike the cultural ideal of slenderness I saw in magazines, movies and virtually every other media channel. As the number I saw on my bathroom scale went up, my sense of self-worth plummeted. During this period of my life, it was rare for me to appreciate and value any of my other qualities—my sense of humor, my loving heart, my intelligence or my creative talent. All of these qualities became secondary in comparison to my weight. I believed the voice in my head that often told me that *who* I was wasn't nearly as important as what I weighed. I had no idea I could ignore that voice if I wanted to, or even silence it altogether.

On top of being angry with myself for what I perceived as my lack of self-control, I was also incredibly angry with my body. I believed it was my body's fault that I had gained so much weight. I felt it had betrayed me by "making" me eat, and so it became the chief target of my hostility. It never occurred to me that my body was the victim of the emotional appetites I was attempting to feed with food. I didn't know that my body was a physical expression of the turmoil I carried deep inside. Each time I looked in the mirror and saw evidence of what I believed were my physical flaws, I blamed my body for it, relentlessly picking out all the ways it didn't live up to my expectations. The remorse and dislike for what I saw when I looked in the bathroom mirror only further eroded my self-esteem.

In my desperation to "get my old body back," the healthy and athletic one I'd taken for granted when I was a teenager, I tried every weight-reduction method imaginable. I gained and lost hundreds of pounds over the years, trying so many diets and diet products that I could officially be listed in The Dieter's Hall of Fame. Sticking to a restricted diet of any kind was incredibly difficult for me. When I did manage to stay on one, I'd end up losing a few pounds, but none of the weight ever stayed off for long. Rather it came back at warp speed, along with a few extra bonus pounds.

After umpteen unsuccessful efforts to lose weight through dieting, I had to begrudgingly admit to myself that diets were not working for me. In fact, I finally realized that they seemed to be working *against* me. The question that then plagued me was, "Well, if diets *don't* work, what the $#%@&* does?"

Out of sheer anguish, I embarked upon a personal experiential research project in which I was the guinea pig, to discover, once and for all, the healthiest, most effective and most enjoyable way to lose excess weight…and keep it off. I threw myself into the research unreservedly, reading anything I could get my hands on that I thought might help me to meet my goal of "losing" extra weight. (I now refer to it almost exclusively as "releasing" excess weight because "losing" anything doesn't sound as empowered or appealing.) I surfed the net for information, sought the help of a therapist, attended dozens of seminars, joined support groups and started working with a personal coach. I was relentless, voracious and passionate in my quest. I even went so far as to approach people in passing who were in great shape to find out their secret to looking so fit.

After all the data was in, I was surprised to find out that it was my body, the one I had been judging so harshly for so many years, that would provide the key to releasing all of the weight I had gained through overeating! It was an epiphany that served me powerfully. Ironically, my *lack* of awareness of its extraordinary value had prevented me from understanding that my body could offer me far more wisdom than I'd ever find in any diet book. I realized I'd been drowning out the one qualified voice that could lead me directly to my natural, ideal weight. So I began to listen.

As I reviewed my own history in terms of my relationship with my body, it became obvious to me that my progressive judgments toward my body paralleled the intensity of my compulsion with food. I was far more likely to want to eat a candy bar (or twenty) after looking in the mirror and judging my appearance harshly. When I was *mentally* down, I was far more likely to *chow* down. In other words, the more I judged my body *and* myself for overeating, the more I ate and the more weight I gained. Judging myself in order to get motivated to lose weight was like shooting myself in the foot before the finals of a dance competition. It was supremely foolish, destructive and self-sabotaging.

The realization that "Body Judgment = Compulsive Eating" didn't come as a complete surprise, but somehow breaking it down to this simple equation deepened my understanding of what I needed to do to break the cycle. If I wanted to achieve my natural weight, the weight at which I would experience optimum health and energy, the *first* thing I had to do was stop judging my body, and myself, so unfairly and unkindly.

It took me a long time to stop judging my body and even longer to start loving it. I didn't have a "body love manual" to follow, and my long-standing belief that I was most attractive when I was super-lean was deeply imbedded. But I stayed committed to treating my body in a more loving way (exercising, choosing predominantly healthy foods, taking vitamins, getting enough rest and limiting my negative thoughts about it), and consequently my emotional appetites diminished and excess weight began to disappear.

With each passing year, I have reached deeper levels of friendship with my body. It no longer feels like a huge burden, but rather an extraordinarily generous gift from the Universe. Instead of repeatedly experiencing daily food hangovers that leave me feeling sick and exhausted, my body now feels healthy, excited, energetic and alive. And that, my friend, is what is in store for you!

I have maintained my natural weight for over ten years now, with only minor fluctuations. This feels phenomenal. What feels even *better*, however, is the fact that I live free from my intense compulsion around food. On a scale of 1 to 10, I would say that my compulsion was once at a 10 plus, and it is now a mere .05. I wake up in the morning without immediately thinking of eating, or of the boring foods I am restricted to on the latest diet I am trying, or how self-conscious I am about my how my body looks. I no longer have the urge to binge eat, having finally learned how to nurture myself and breathe through difficult feelings. I thoroughly enjoy eating without feeling guilty or worried that I'm going to return to my old compulsive eating patterns. I couldn't eat at that old level of compulsion even if I wanted to. Now *that's* the ultimate freedom!

Understandably, after my long and painful struggle with compulsive eating and body shame, the connected, accepting and appreciative relationship I have with my body today is a deeply treasured gift. The time I have devoted to loving my body has provided me with benefits far above and beyond reaching my natural weight. Perhaps most importantly, I have learned to value myself independent of how I look, and I am experiencing peace and happiness on levels I didn't know were available to me.

The Mindful Eating Method will support you as you begin to shift from being critical of your body *and* yourself, to being deeply appreciative. So that you too can know joy every day, I'm going to share with you *everything* I have learned on my road to recovery. Every perspective, practice and habit that helped me to overcome body rejection and compulsive overeating is now yours.

I recommend taking your time as you read *The Mindful Eating Method*, putting it down periodically and giving yourself time to digest the material offered. It is a book to be revisited again and again, and each time you do so, new insights will come to you.

As we take this journey together, you will learn, as I did, that your body has a language all its own and it communicates to you through your physical *feelings*. You will, with practice, start to decipher your own body's unique language, the specific ways it conveys its limits, needs and preferences to you. As you learn to recognize its specific signals for "hungry" and "satisfied" and to honor those signals consistently, you will naturally release your excess weight without dieting, obsessive exercise, counting calories, taking appetite suppressants or denying yourself *any* of your favorite foods.

I call eating in synchronicity with your physical hunger *"Eating in Alliance"* with your body. There are ten practices in the *Eating in Alliance* program. Following these practices allowed me to overcome my compulsive relationship with food and achieve my natural weight, without dieting or denying myself any of the foods that I love (yeah)! If you follow the guidelines offered in this book, it won't be a question of *if* you are going to achieve your ideal weight; rather it will be a question of *when.*

There will be recommendations for healthy ways to reconnect with your body throughout the book. Experiment with all of them, choose the ones that feel right for you and leave the others behind, for now. You are a unique individual, and ultimately you will add your own stamp of originality to your journey to body love by defining, through experimentation, the specific combination of practices that will allow you to experience peace with food, your body and yourself.

I also offer a thirty-day program in which you can partner with another person who is struggling with their relationship with food so that you can team up and expedite your own healing process. It is not required that you have a partner to work the program. Although it is undeniably easier, it is not a mandatory component. Rather it is an additional asset that will support your intention to reconnect with your body and achieve your natural weight.

Learning to love my own body, and in equal measure, myself, has supported me in creating not only a healthy, beautiful body but also a life that has exceeded my greatest dreams. Through my life experience, I have come to know that love, in its many forms, is the strongest force on earth. If you focus that powerful force on your body, you will break through the confines of food compulsions and body shame and free yourself to experience all the joy life offers. You deserve it. We all do. My intention is to support you in embracing and loving your body, as well as yourself, so that you can live your life in *tremendous* joy with a much greater realization of the sacred and loveable being you are. Welcome to the first page of the rest of your life.

I feel privileged to be a part of your journey.

Lily

*****

"Nothing in the world arouses more false hope than the first four hours of a diet."

–Anonymous

Chapter 1

The Diet Deception

Why Diets Do Not Work!

As I look back on the battle I waged against my body, I have a lot of regrets. One of the biggest is that I subjected my body to an *endless* succession of futile and ineffective diets. Crazy, unhealthy fad diets and "doctor recommended" diets, I tried them all. It took me over a decade to discover what every veteran dieter knows: diets don't work.

These are not the bitter rantings of a woman who couldn't stick to a diet (although Lord knows I couldn't). It is a confirmed fact. Diets fail *ninety-five to ninety-eight percent of the time.* And by fail, I mean that although you may lose weight *initially*, you will inevitably gain it back, and most of us will pick up a few extra pounds along the way. Research indicates that only ten percent of dieters keep the weight off for two years, and just *two* percent keep the weight off for seven years. More than 26,000 diet methods have been published since the 1920s, and yet, with *extremely* rare exception, none provide more than a temporary weight loss. That should be *more* than enough proof that diets are ineffective, and yet the diet mania persists. The fact that diets work *temporarily* is a big part of the problem. Dieters get hooked on the high of their short-term weight loss and this high keeps them coming back again and again *in spite* of the fact that they almost always regain the weight…and then some.

Not only are diets not *helpful*, they are also often tremendously *harmful* in terms of both your emotional and physical well-being. Knowing what I now know after studying and participating in every diet that crossed my desperate path for over a decade, I believe with all of my being that, just as there are health warnings from the Surgeon General on every package of cigarettes, there should be a warning label attached to every diet program which should read: "Danger: Diets are almost always ineffective for long-term weight loss, can create additional weight gain, a deep dive in self-esteem, a hugely compulsive relationship with food and, all too frequently, a full-blown compulsive eating disorder.

I know how emotionally debilitating and dangerous dieting can be from my own painful experience. My unhealthy relationship with food and with my body began my senior year in high school when I went on a diet for the very first time. Prior to then, my relationship with food had been normal and healthy. As a child and throughout most of my teenage years, I ate when my body told me to; I stopped when I felt full, and I rarely thought about food unless I was physically hungry. I ate any and every food that appealed to me, and my energy levels, weight and overall health were great. While I can't say I loved my body the way I do today, back then I truly liked my body and appreciated how it looked.

In my early teens, as my interest in boys developed, I became more preoccupied with how it would appear to others. Like any typical teenager, my desire to be attractive to the opposite sex intensified. *Seventeen* magazine, which I used to devour whenever I got my hands on it, featured *exceptionally* lean young models and almost *always* included the most recent diet trend. Although no one came right out and said it, I still got the message loud, clear and in stereo: Thin was beautiful, sexy and desirable. I didn't see any full-figured girls in the magazine, so the assumption I made was that full figures were simply not as attractive as lean ones.

As I was slowly indoctrinated into this cultural perspective, I started stepping on the scale every day to make sure I wasn't putting on extra pounds. A mild, but slowly escalating paranoia started to develop, but my weight stayed steady throughout high school, up until my senior year. At that time, many of my friends were already dieting, or at least closely watching what they ate. Boneless, skinless chicken breasts, fruit, vegetables and green salads with low-fat dressing or no dressing at all, became staple meals for many of them. At just over five feet, six inches and weighing in at one hundred sixteen pounds, I had no legitimate need to worry about my weight. But because there was so much emphasis on being thin at my school, within my own family, among many of my friends, and in American culture at large, I gradually found myself

15

joining the ranks of those who were overly obsessed with being thin.

I remember with total clarity the circumstances that prompted me to go on my very first diet. It was almost at the end of my senior year and a handsome, sweet college freshman named Peter had asked me out on a date. I had a huge crush on him and when he invited me to go to the beach with some of his college friends, I was thrilled beyond belief. I went out the very next day to buy a new swimsuit, so I could be absolutely sure I looked my best. I remember choosing a one-piece suit with soft pastel rainbow stripes and a matching belt. The suit was adorable. But as I examined myself in the dressing room mirror, under the full glare of the unforgiving lights that changing rooms are notorious for, I started to compare my shorter, more athletic figure to those of the super- lean and tall girls I had seen in movies and fashion magazines. I felt my reflection fell short of their kind of beauty, and an awful feeling of insecurity washed over me. As I stared at my mirror image, my judgments began to snowball as I found other reasons to pick at myself. Suddenly, as though I had donned cultural spectacles, I saw my breasts as too small and my thighs as too full, with far too much cellulite. I can remember grimacing at my reflection and thinking, "I need to lose weight and firm up these *jiggly* legs, and *fast*."

I changed back into my clothes, went out to the cash register and paid for the swimsuit, but my enthusiasm about the beach date was deflated like a bounce house at the end of a county fair because I was so worried about how I would look. I went straight home from the shopping center, stepped on the scale and saw that I was, in fact, a few pounds over my usual weight. That number, one hundred eighteen pounds, depressed me for the rest of the day. Oh, the insanity of it all!

I started to worry that if my date saw me in the bright light of day in my swimsuit, he would no longer find me attractive. Absurdly, those few pounds made me feel so unworthy and inadequate that they impacted my *entire* state of mind. It no longer mattered to me that I was kind, smart, funny or creative. All of my self-esteem was suddenly wrapped up in how my body looked—or how I *thought* it looked. Sadly, it never occurred to me that Peter would be *far* more focused on what *was* attractive about me than he would be on my "flaws." *I* became so obsessed with my weight that I projected that *he* would be, too. Ridiculous, yes of course, but only in retrospect. At the time, that was my reality and you would have been hard-pressed to talk me out of it.

With only two days before my big date, I decided I to go on a crash diet. I chose an all-vegetable diet, which I had read in one of my teen magazines was one of the fastest ways to lose weight. I didn't know the first thing about cooking, so I basically ate canned and pre-cooked Del Monte string beans for two days straight. In my heart and in my body, dieting felt *completely* unnatural from the start. I felt anxious, fussy and uncomfortable. Normally a happy teenager, I was cranky and out of sorts for those two days. I began to intensely crave and obsess over the foods I would be able to eat when I finished my diet. I couldn't wait! Instead of looking forward to being with Peter for a fun day at the beach, I was now excitedly anticipating the *end* of the date so I could eat what I wanted once again.

I did manage to diet myself down to one hundred sixteen pounds before the date, but that didn't last long. The day after the date I went on a massive eating binge. Having denied myself regular food for just two days, my eating patterns became distorted and unnatural. I regained the two pounds I had lost on the diet, plus an additional two pounds the following week.

That summer, after I graduated from high school, I became even more obsessed with getting thin. Because I was leaving for college and wanted to feel confident at my new school, I dieted constantly, and then, in reaction to the deprivation, I began to binge regularly.

In late September I packed my bags and left for college at Santa Clara University. My transition to college was *far* more challenging than I had anticipated and brought on an entirely new level of stress that I definitely wasn't equipped to handle. While it was exciting to be living away from home for the first time, it was also intimidating. I was insecure and immature in many ways. The college lifestyle was far less structured than the one I had at home, and I struggled to find a balance between meeting the academic demands and enjoying my new freedom. The new pressures *and* my lack of coping mechanisms added to my already significant obsession with food.

Unlike living at home, there were virtually *no* rules in college. I could eat whenever and whatever I wanted, stay up as late as I chose and pretty much do whatever I pleased without anyone watching. The lack of boundaries, though fun in many respects, did not serve me well. Instead of the three square meals my mom had almost always prepared for me, I had *unlimited* access to dormitory meals. I started using food, especially breads, candy, cookies, ice cream and rich desserts to relax, nurture and comfort myself. During my freshman year I gained about twenty-five pounds, a common tradition among first-year female students that was known affectionately as "Benson Butt" in reference to Benson Hall (where the cafeteria was located). The more weight I gained, the more fanatical I became about losing it. I became a dieting maniac, so obsessed with my weight that I would jump on the scale two to three times a day.

As if my relationship with food wasn't already dysfunctional enough, one late night a close girlfriend pulled me aside after we had polished off a pizza together and introduced me to her weight-control method, purging. I *despised* purging from the first time I tried it. It totally grossed me out, but my desperation to lose weight overrode my disgust. After I added purging to my bingeing, I began an even deeper descent into my imbalanced relationship with food. Between the purging and dieting, my body must have felt like it was under attack.

I was a typical yo-yo dieter, getting into a pattern in which I'd gain two pounds, lose two pounds, gain five pounds, lose two, gain fifteen more, and on and on it went. Those who have experienced compulsivity around food know that psychologically and physically, food for a compulsive overeater is *every* bit as irresistible as a drink to an alcoholic or a fix for a drug addict. It was crazy, even to myself, that almost every thought I had seemed to be about food: when I was going to eat, how much I was going to eat, and even where I was going to eat without being watched. I could have completed my Master's degree, gotten a Ph.D. and learned to play the tuba with all the time I spent worrying about my weight and thinking about food.

Post-college, with each passing year, my addiction intensified and my weight continued to climb. In total desperation, I experimented with dangerous diet drugs, laxatives and diuretics. For months on end, I would binge and purge at least twice a day. Not surprisingly, I experienced many of the dangerous side effects that accompany all of these unhealthy choices, including disorientation, diarrhea, heart arrhythmia, shaking, nausea, dehydration and exhaustion. Too embarrassed to expose my eating problem to even my closest friends or family members, I silently rationalized my behavior. I was more afraid of being overweight than anything I could think of, and I would do, and did, almost anything to be thin. I lost sight of how precious my health was and my ability to see almost any good in myself was shattered.

My negative body image and lack of self-esteem made life's ordinary challenges seem *much* bigger. Small inconveniences were blown out of proportion, and I would turn to food to turn the volume down on my intense emotions. If I was frustrated or stressed for any reason—about work, relationships, an upcoming test or a traffic jam—I would head to the kitchen and reach for a treat in an attempt to curb my angst. The food never reduced my emotional discomfort for more than a short while, and it left me with the added burden of guilt and self-condemnation for overeating. It seems crazy now, but I just didn't know any other way to take care of myself at the time.

Over the years, I gained and lost hundreds of pounds, my weight fluctuating between one hundred and sixteen and one hundred and eighty pounds. Even when I had a temporary success and came close to reaching my goal weight, I could not fully enjoy the results because I was still utterly fixated on food. Additionally, I lived with the constant worry that I would regain my weight. No matter what the scale said, I was never really satisfied with the way I looked and was often envious of girls who looked thinner and who appeared to maintain their figures effortlessly.

As I look back on those years, I can remember feeling incredibly frightened, lonely and isolated in my addiction. I used to lie awake at night and wonder if I was going to end up accidentally killing myself from the variety of ways I was abusing my body. I had read about the growing number of deaths related to bulimia as well as the appetite suppressants and diuretics I was taking. Those years were the most challenging of my life, and it is still very painful to recall how poorly I treated my body and myself.

I am well aware that my story is not unique. I wish it were. But the fact is that millions of women, and now an increasing number of men and girls, are living with their own painful version of my struggle. Tragically, chronic dieting is now considered normal behavior. Women *and* men are starving themselves and following diet regimens that have little to do with being healthy and everything to do with losing weight as quickly as possible. Shockingly, it is *still* not common or accepted knowledge that diets don't work and there are many people who believe, as I did, that they are alone in their inability to stick to a diet.

At one point, I didn't *want* to believe that diets didn't work. I can remember telling myself, "It has been my lack of self-control, not the diet, that prevented me from losing weight." I rationalized, "I just haven't found the *right* diet for me." Part of me must have fought against realizing that if I accepted that diets *didn't* work, I would be admitting I had spent close to a decade using a flawed approach. I didn't want to be wrong about something I had invested so much time and energy in. Somehow it felt safer to stay with what was familiar, even though it wasn't working and it was making me miserable. As crazy as that seems to me in retrospect, I was so consumed by that way of living that I simply could not see clearly. I clung to my dieter's mentality like a hungry baby clings to its mother's bosom.

Gradually, I began to see and accept that the devil I knew (dieting) was preventing me from getting over my obsession with food *and* was keeping me from releasing my excess weight. My history with dieting was the best proof of that. As I became more willing to let go of dieting and instead explore a whole new way of relating to food and my body, the doors to the mental cell I had created for myself swung open and I was freed, just as you will be. Self-imposed prisons are sometimes the most challenging to break out of, but when you choose to unlock the door *yourself*, the sense of liberation is indescribably wonderful. Releasing yourself from the dieter's mentality is an important step in your journey.

You probably know from your own years of dieting and innumerable failed weight-loss attempts that diets don't work. Even so, in the face of ubiquitous radio, television and magazine advertisements that make seductive weight-loss promises, you might find that it feels almost impossible to resist the impulse to take yet another stab at the latest "breakthrough" program or product, only to be devastated when you regain the weight and then some. The difficulty of breaking this cycle (and indeed perhaps even an addiction to dieting itself) is why we need to take a little time to understand *exactly* why diets don't work.

The Physical Reasons Why Diets Don't Work

During my extensive weight-release research project, I learned that the most basic reason that diets don't work is that they run counter to your body's most basic survival instincts. What do I mean by that? Well, in the days of our earliest ancestors, there were no guarantees that they would be able to feed themselves and their families. Instead, there were times of feasting and times of famine. When food was abundant (summer and spring) everyone ate well. In the lean times—during winter when it was difficult to hunt, gather or grow food, or when drought, flood or vermin wiped out food supplies—people survived on what little they could find and the few items they could store, such as nuts and root vegetables.

Our ancestors avoided starving to death because their bodies helped them to adapt to severe shortages of food. How? By storing fat more efficiently in part through slowing down the *metabolism* (i.e., the rate at which the body burns calories) so that it simply did not require as much food to survive.

So what does that have to do with dieting? Everything! Your body interprets a diet as a famine. Every time you restrict your food intake, your body goes into *survival* mode, slowing your metabolism because it thinks that, by doing so, it is ensuring your survival!

As you can see, diets work overtime against your efforts to release excess weight. Current statistics show that after only one diet, your metabolism can slow by as much as forty percent. *Forty percent*! Furthermore, it can take up to a year for your metabolism to return to its pre-diet calorie-burning capacity! This metabolic slowdown would explain why people tend to gain *more* weight back after a diet, typically around ten percent.

Here's how the metabolic meltdown might work in your case. Let's say you weigh one hundred sixty pounds and you normally burn 2,000 calories a day. You start a diet that restricts you to only 1,100 calories a day. Your body, recognizing that it is getting far fewer calories than normal, interprets this as *starvation* because it doesn't understand that you are *intentionally* reducing your food intake. It then *purposefully* starts reducing the number of calories necessary to keep you functioning by *lowering* your metabolism (slowing down the rate at which you burn calories). That way it can help you "survive" on the small portions you are eating.

Let's say after a few weeks on a diet, you manage to make it to the end (no small miracle) and you drop ten pounds. Now you go off the diet and start to eat what was, before the diet, normal for you. Unfortunately, your body has now adjusted to 1,100 calories a day by lowering your metabolism. When you go back to eating 2,000 calories a day, in the worst-case scenario, your metabolic rate has dropped forty percent! Your body now thinks it is getting an *excess* 900 calories, which it will then store and hoard as fat. So, when you return to your regular eating habits, not only will you gain back the ten pounds, but you may also put on a few more. And, if you are one of the unlucky forty percent, it could take up to a *year* for your body to recognize that the "famine" is over and raise your metabolism back up to the pre-diet rate! Yikes! That explains a lot, doesn't it? No wonder dieting and losing weight has been such a struggle! All the physical discomfort and emotional frustration of dieting is wasted because the temporary weight loss achieved is frequently offset by the long-term damage done by a lowered metabolic rate.

And these virtually unquestionable arguments against dieting represent only the *physical* side of the story. There are equally valid and inarguable psychological reasons why diets are predestined to fail.

The Psychological Reasons Why Diets Don't Work

Diets are mentally disempowering in part because they are so restrictive *and* because your dieter's mentality overrides your willingness to pay attention to your body's communications. Your body says, "I want to eat. I'm really hungry and I'm feeling like I need some carbohydrates for energy." But your dieter's mind says, "No, you've already had your allotment for the day. Have a celery stick if you are hungry."

The diet becomes like a very strict parent trying to control a child's natural appetites, like the mother who says, "Don't eat that, wait until dinner!" even when you are *really* hungry. Dieting sets you up to experience an immature psychological state of powerlessness much like the one we may have experienced in childhood when our parent(s) had control over so much of our lives. In the course of their development, children fight against not being able to make their own choices by testing limits, pleading, whining, sulking and even throwing tantrums. Without adequate opportunities to make decisions for themselves, they rebel against being overly controlled. It is part of their becoming individuals, and they'll fight for their independence, even when it means breaking the rules. They'll even sneak and tell lies to experience autonomy. Now fast-forward to adulthood and the model of dieting with its tight food restrictions, which can make you feel confined both physically and mentally. It's only reasonable to expect that you will feel frustrated and powerless and it's equally reasonable to expect that you, too, will rebel.

Psychologically, the deprivation of dieting causes a reaction that Neal Barnard, M.D., calls the "restrained eater phenomenon." In his book, *The Power of Your Plate*, Dr. Barnard states that when we deprive ourselves of food, even by choice, the physical and emotional stress can lead to emotional roller coasters, low self-esteem and irrational behavior (like eating when you're not hungry). So, when your body tells you it is hungry and you ignore the cues because you are attempting to stay on a diet, your mind will fixate on the food you are withholding, like the child who has been told not to touch the presents underneath the Christmas tree. It follows that a restricted diet virtually *ensures* that you will be emotionally and psychologically drawn to doing what you (the restrictive "parent") have told yourself (the hungry "child") you must not do. It is not surprising, then, that children who are put on diets are *far* more likely to binge than children who are allowed to eat according to their own healthy appetites.

No matter what your age, there is a childlike aspect to who you are, which is often referred to as an "inner child." *Healthy* expressions of the inner child include being silly, spontaneous, carefree, adventurous, curious, imaginative and playful. *Wounded* aspects of your inner child include a sense of powerlessness, rebelliousness, defensiveness, hurt, guilt, irrationality, confusion, impulsivity, insecurity and fear. These wounded child qualities are usually over-amplified in people who didn't feel safe, loved or appreciated in their childhood or who experienced some form of insensitivity, neglect or emotional or physical abuse.

It is in large part your wounded inner child's worries, fears and self-doubts that stimulate the uncomfortable feelings you attempt to avoid by eating compulsively. In many cases, the more challenging your childhood, the more a negative and disempowering voice can dominate your thoughts about yourself and your life circumstances. Oftentimes, the harder your parents were on you as a child, the harder you will be on yourself as an adult. How does this relate to dieting? Well, somewhere in the midst of your diet when you eat more than you think you should, you become your own angry parent. You punish yourself with self-judgments like a frustrated parent would punish a disobedient child.

For many years I couldn't see that judging myself harshly, without understanding or compassion, was a form of self-abuse. Although I knew that allowing someone else to treat me unkindly and unfairly was most certainly self-destructive, I didn't know that when I internalized my self-judgment and was unkind to myself, it was every bit as debilitating. When you judge *yourself* for going off your diet rather than laying blame on the true culprit—the diet itself—it is like punishing a child for an innocent mistake. *Dieting* is the problem, not you!

The fact is that dieting prevents you from learning to trust your own body. Like a child being forced to eat whatever is being served, even if they hate it, a diet impedes your ability to make selections based upon what your body *truly* wants and needs. Your body may need protein in the morning when the diet calls for fruit. You may be best served by eating a bowl of oatmeal upon waking when instead you are eating the recommended eggs and bacon. Your appetites are unique to you alone, and only *you* and your body know what food choices are most appropriate on any given day. Blanket diet programs simply can't fit every body's unique and varying requirements.

If you have been struggling with your relationship with food for a while, you may have lost confidence in your ability to decide *what* to eat and *when* to eat it. You might find it somewhat comforting to follow a diet program exactly as it is written, rather than facing the uncertainty of choosing from unlimited food options over and over again each day. But if you're like me—and like most people who've ever dieted—after the initial rush of starting a new structured program, you soon find yourself frustrated by the restrictions of the plan, and a backlash occurs. That may involve a momentary lapse where you eat a few things off your diet, going on a free-for-all binge in the middle of it, or giving up entirely on the program out of pure frustration.

Fortunately there's a middle ground. There's a way to develop a new approach to eating that recognizes your unique preferences and needs, within a framework that will help you keep your choices on track. We'll discuss this in detail in Chapter 6 (*"Eating in Alliance* with Your Body"). For now, just start to consider the possibility that you *and* your body have the wisdom to choose foods that are right for you, that will allow you to reach and maintain your ideal weight *without* relying on a restricted menu dictated by someone other than you. My intention is to support you in developing a connected relationship with your body that will allow you the freedom to eat *any* type of food your body physically craves. A healthy connection with your body and a true understanding of its needs will support you in learning to differentiate your physical hungers from your emotional hungers, so that you can take back your power, choose the food that's right for you and let go of the self-sabotaging rebellion that we all resort to when dieting.

Diets Don't Address the Root of the Problem

Finally, a significant reason that diets don't result in permanent weight loss is because they don't address the *real* cause of excess weight—your emotional issues and their related hungers. Any time you eat for reasons other than physical hunger, you are most likely attempting to escape uncomfortable emotions such as fear, worry, anger, sadness, tension, confusion or boredom (or even pleasurable emotions that are rare for you). Alternately, you might be using food as a way to generate a *positive* emotion such as pleasure, calmness, satisfaction or happiness.

"Escape eating" is most common among compulsive eaters because most of us don't know how to deal with intense and uncomfortable feelings. It takes being curious, patient and courageous to face and cope with your full range of emotions. As members of the human race, we are all hard-wired to seek pleasure and avoid pain. We're all joy junkies at heart, so dealing with the messiness of some of our emotions is *really* unappealing. Given that we'd rather feel good than *anything* else, it is frequently easier to head to the refrigerator to find something to fill up that unpleasant or empty place inside. But eating when you are not hungry in order to make yourself feel better is like pumping air into a leaky tire again and again, rather than finding the *holes* where the air is escaping and patching *them*. By overeating, you are attempting to deal with the symptoms of the problem (uncomfortable feelings) instead of the root cause (emotional hungers).

One thing's for certain. There isn't a diet in the world that will patch those leaks, and we've already seen the damage that dieting does to your body and your psyche. In order to break the bingeing cycle, one of the keys is exploring the specific reasons you eat when you are not physically hungry. It will take more than a burger and fries to heal an emotional wound, and the sooner you identify the "leaks" in your life, the faster you can patch them and be on your merry way. Farther along in the book, we will explore the *specific* issues that often lie at the heart of compulsive eating and address specific *beliefs* that fuel compulsive eating habits. You'll get to the root of why it is so difficult for you to process certain emotions and you'll learn techniques to ride the wave of the difficult ones until they dissipate, like an ocean wave does when it

30

hits the shore.

Final Warning: Diets and Diet Pills Can Be Deadly

My own brush with the potentially fatal side effects of dieting came from taking the prescription diet pill and appetite suppressant Fen-Phen. At the time I was only about twenty-five pounds over my natural weight, and as usual, I was looking for a quick way to lose it. I found my answer on a walk with my friend Carrie. She had started taking Fen-Phen, had lost about ten pounds and looked great. Impressed with *her* rapid weight loss and desperate to do the same, I made an appointment to see her doctor. As I waited in the examination room, I was hoping the appointment wouldn't take too long because I had another commitment across town. I needn't have worried. The doctor was in and out of the room so fast it made my head spin. He gave me a prescription for Fen-Phen after only an extremely cursory review of the medical history sheet I had filled out and after quickly eyeballing my body. However, I was *thrilled* to have a new diet pill to try. Surely, I thought, *this* will be the trick that gets me down to my goal weight once and for all. Then I'll start eating healthier foods and working out more. (How familiar does that story sound?)

I took the recommended daily dosage and sure enough, my appetite was radically diminished, and I started releasing weight. But the doctor neglected to tell me there would be a number of *overwhelming* side effects. Perhaps if I had been warned in advance that I would begin to feel my heart beating as if I had just run a marathon, I wouldn't have been so alarmed when it happened. Maybe if I had realized I was going

31

to feel extremely agitated and edgy, like I had just downed about ten cups of coffee, I would not have taken the pills in the first place. Maybe if the doctor himself had known that there were some women who had died of complications after taking Fen-Phen, he wouldn't have written out my prescription with such nonchalance. In spite of my body rejecting the drug, I soldiered on in desperation. When I finished my first bottle of pills I had lost about thirteen pounds, which predictably, I promptly regained once I went off the drug and went back to a normal eating regime. I called the doctor and asked for another prescription, which he gave me without even asking to see me again or asking about my well being.

I later found out that Fen-Phen was an amphetamine, essentially "speed." At that time the long-term effects of this drug and its potentially fatal side effects were not widely reported, so I had no way of knowing I was risking my life to lose weight. I also didn't know that obesity researchers had discovered that Fen-Phen causes brain damage in laboratory animals, destroying the neural axons that produce serotonin, the calming, feel-good chemical in the brain, the very one that makes you feel happy. Once I found out Fen-Phen could potentially kill off the very chemical that made me feel good *permanently*, and, even more frighteningly, could be fatal, I decided to flush the remainder of my new prescription of diet drugs down the toilet. I vividly remember staring at the two dozen or so brightly colored yellow pills swirling around the bottom of the white porcelain bowl.

That flush was a strong statement to myself that I was no longer willing to risk my health, let alone my life, to be thin. It was also an important step in my learning to trust my own judgment rather than handing off my choices about food and my body to someone else—not even a doctor. Trusting my body was and continues to be one of the smartest choices I have ever made. When you do the same, you will connect with a powerful resource that will enable you to transform your relationship with food – for good.

In Laura Fraser's powerful expose of the diet industry she wrote, "Although every diet may not lead to an eating disorder, almost every eating disorder begins with a diet." I know my own compulsive relationship with food was *unquestioningly* set off by my first diet attempt, perhaps you will find upon reflection that the same is true for you.

The National Association of Anorexia Nervosa and Associated Disorders estimates that eight million Americans suffer from either anorexia or bulimia, both of which can result in very serious medical problems, even death. Treatment for anorexia and bulimia are beyond the scope of this book, but if you're struggling with an illness of that kind, I have listed a number of resources at the end of this book (Appendix A) to support your healing. As I mentioned in Chapter 1, I suffered from bulimia for many years. If I could go back and do it over again I would have gotten help much earlier. As soon as I saw myself sliding down the slippery slope of an eating disorder, I would have begun to look for a competent therapist who would support me in my recovery as soon as possible, and I encourage you to do the same. Eating disorders typically get progressively worse, so take it *very* seriously, and do not underestimate the danger to your health. Be brave and make a phone call. Honor yourself by taking the bold step of asking for help.

Getting to the Heart of the Matter

Throughout the book I offer what I call "Awareness Opportunities." These are exercises specifically designed to bring you into deeper relationship with yourself and your body. You may be tempted to gloss over them, to answer them briefly in your mind and move on quickly. I wanted to do the same when I was reading many a self-help book, to take the short cut because it seemed boring or inconvenient to spend time with the questions. But the growth comes when you dive into the questions with your full heart and mind. Don't shortchange yourself by taking the easy route. Push yourself beyond your comfort zone and allow yourself to see each question as an opportunity to know your *self* on a more intimate level. The deeper the questions you ask yourself, the more your self-awareness will grow. Writing your answers stimulates all sorts of new understanding. You access a part of your mind (the subconscious) that stores memories that might have been long forgotten or others that are only vague recollections. If you give your all to each Awareness Opportunity, it will support your intention to love your body and yourself and thereby release your excess weight, which is, after all, why you're reading this book. You can use a beautiful leather-bound journal or a plain old spiral notebook, but get yourself something to write with and let's get started.

Awareness Opportunity

Take a moment and review your dieting history. If you need to, Google the word "diet" or "appetite suppressant" to jog your memory about the diets and diet products you've tried. Briefly answer the following questions for each:

What diets have you tried?

How did the diet (product) make you feel when you were on it?

How much weight did you lose on the diet(s)?

How much weight did you gain back?

After reviewing your history, how do you feel about dieting today?

Now that you have a stronger understanding of why diets *don't* work, it is time to explore what *does*. The saying "Insanity is doing the same thing over and over again and expecting a different result" has been attributed to various sources, including Benjamin Franklin, Albert Einstein and old Chinese proverbs. Regardless of who said it originally, when put in the context of dieting, *it is time to end the insanity*. It's time to try the *sane* approach, one that actually allows you to release excess weight! The next chapter explores one of the primary relationships that will support you in doing just that.

*****

"To love oneself is the beginning of a life-long romance."

-Oscar Wilde

Chapter 2

Loving Yourself

The Fast Track to Achieving Your Ideal Weight

Given the complicated nature of compulsive eating issues, there are *multiple* purposes for this book. One is to support you in freeing yourself from a compulsive relationship with food while you develop a healthy and harmonious relationship with your body. Another is to assist you in developing a more loving relationship with the person who lives *inside* that body–YOU–wonderful, complicated, lovable, perfectly imperfect and extraordinary you! The second purpose (loving yourself) supports the first (overcoming compulsive eating) because the more you love and appreciate yourself, the happier, more whole and "full" you will feel, which in turn makes it *much* easier to overcome the urge to eat when you are not hungry.

Believe it or not, love (specifically loving yourself and loving your body) is a crucial key to releasing excess weight. You've heard the old adage

"Love conquers all." Well, it's true. Not only does it conquer all, but it *heals* all as well. It brings ecstasy, relieves pain, opens hearts, produces clarity, creates unity, cures illness, dispels loneliness, drives out illusions, reveals the truth, moves mountains and brings light to the darkness. Love, simply stated, is a one-stop joy shop! Can I get an AMEN!

It is the essence of your heart and the answer to your woes. Love possesses many facets ranging from the soft, gentle love you offer when tender feelings are hurt, to the strong and firm love that requires setting limits and boundaries for yourself so you can overcome old, unhealthy habits. Love is generous, forgiving, creative and wise.

Love is not only an extraordinarily powerful and versatile energy, it is in fact the *strongest* energy in existence, which is why, when you extend it to yourself, it has the capacity to transform your life in astounding ways. In the words of Dr. Martin Luther King, Jr., "I know that love is ultimately the only answer to mankind's problems, and I'm going to talk about it everywhere I go." The effects of love, when directed at yourself, will happily stun you. Self-love, when practiced with consistency, supports you in creating your own "inner sanctuary" where you feel safe, loved and calm. You trust that regardless of what is happening in your life, you can count on *yourself* to nurture, honor, love and take care of yourself, both physically and mentally. From this empowered place your fear and worry diminish, as do your emotional appetites.

The joy that accompanies having a loving relationship with myself has filled me in a way that no food, no matter how delicious, possibly could.

My self-love not only healed my relationship with my body, but my emotional hungers for acceptance, fulfillment, joy, safety and peace as well. The internal healing is now reflected in my healthy body. Because I have learned to soothe myself *internally* through self-loving thoughts and behaviors, it lessened my compulsive *external* attempts to soothe myself through food.

My journey into self-love required a lot of deep contemplation and a passionate and open-minded search for an antidote to my lack of self-appreciation. My journey was not a direct path, but rather a labyrinth. This was in part because I didn't have a model of self-love to follow. I didn't know anyone personally who was in a wholly loving relationship with themselves, so I couldn't ask them how to achieve it. I had read some books that touched on the concept of self-love, but in my daily life, it was *really* hard to practice.

My path included journeying deep into my own soul, which I had read somewhere held all the answers to my problems. I started by exploring my personal history to see how it had impacted my present reality and I started pondering the bigger questions about my life and myself. Instead of wondering what I was going to eat that day, or what diet I was going to go on, I instead asked myself why it was so hard to make choices that I knew were good for me and why I was so hard on myself. I contemplated for the first time my purpose in life and who was I above and beyond my physical being. As I asked myself the deeper questions, my awareness expanded. As I started to explore the beliefs I had that were preventing me from being happy, I was able to break free of negative "thinking" habits that kept me stuck in a mental rut. As I became more comfortable with, and accepting of, myself, I *slowly* stopped using food to numb my feelings, and instead used my feelings to help me figure out where I needed to raise the bar in my physical and emotional life. It was during the course of this journey that I began to have a better understanding of the nature of life and truly began to grasp the extraordinary preciousness and inherent lovability of *all* human beings, including myself.

So what's to love about you? Where to begin... Well, let's start with the fact that you are divine. You were brought into this world as an incredibly adorable, sacred, whole and beautiful soul, an incomparable miracle, and that is what you remain today. Are you always trying to make better choices, to be a better person in some way, to do kind things for others? Those intentions *alone* identify your core goodness, the true objectives of your heart and soul, even when you aren't able to follow through on your best intentions. You are good. I am good. We are all fundamentally good. Not infallible or perfect, mind you, but inherently sacred nonetheless.

Not *only* are you a divine individual, but you are also a member of an incredibly special species. As a member of the human race, you are, by your very nature, an astonishing creature, unique among all life forms, the concoction of the brilliant-beyond-description source that created this planet, our galaxy and the other one hundred billion galaxies (or more) beyond ours. (How's that for a mind bender!) The fact that you were chosen to be a member of the human race and that you get to live

40

on arguably the most beautiful planet in the galaxy, confirms your special place in the cosmos. You have only to compare our lush, life-sustaining planet, filled with a massive array of fascinating plant and animal life to all the other semi-barren, lifeless planets to realize how truly special we are. Our planet is the Ferrari of planets, and we, its blessed inhabitants, are the intergalactic lottery winners. Spend a weekend on Mars and you'll see *exactly* what I mean. You and I were hand picked by the Divine to have a human experience on this miraculous planet.

You are a loveable member of the human race, a holy being. Can you identify on any level with that statement? You may feel like describing yourself in such a reverent way feels too over the top, too self-aggrandizing. I can understand that initial reluctance. If you are hard on yourself as a rule, and embarrassed about some of your current behaviors and past choices, it would be challenging to go from feeling inadequate or unlovable to feeling like a sacred being overnight. That's quite a mental jump for almost anyone, *especially* when your eye has been trained on your perceived inadequacies and big boo-boos for your entire life.

However, the miraculous, divine nature of your existence on this planet is true even if you have made some really poor choices in your life. You may think ill of yourself because you have thought, said or done terrible things, hurt people you loved or been dishonest. Well, my friend, welcome to the human condition.

A word about what I mean when I refer to "The Divine." Throughout the world there are a wide variety of interpretations of, and names for a higher power. Some refer to it as God, some as Buddha, some as Mother Nature, others as Allah, Spirit, Krishna, Christ, Mohammed, Gaia, Source, Mother/Father, Universe, Consciousness, Spirit, Truth, the Tao, Presence, the Creator and the list goes on. For the sake of simplicity, I will use the term "the Divine" to encompass all of these expressions of an unconditionally loving energy. This is with respect for all people and their individual faiths.

We have *all* had thoughts that are horrid. We all have done things of which we are ashamed. We have all made a variety of mistakes, both large and small. It is simply part of the human evolutionary process. We humans are sacred, but still emotionally immature in some ways, which spawns our less-than-ideal traits and actions.

But because we often believe we are one of the only ones who think and behave in a wide variety of these "low-vibration" ways, we are ashamed of ourselves and attempt to hide our humanness from others. We think, "If so-and-so *really* knew what I had done or what I was thinking, if they *really* knew my dark side, they would want nothing to do with me." In reality if we all admitted our humanness, we would be liberated from the erroneous, unbearably lonely notion that we alone have problems, insecurities or a dark side. We are all equally human and judging ourselves for it only gives the "dark" side more power. (Just ask any *Star Wars* fan.)

So how does this relate to overcoming compulsive eating habits? Well, as I discovered on my investigative process, repeated feelings of guilt, shame and inadequacy *stimulate* the emotional hungers that drive you to binge eat. In other words, the weight of your self-judgment is ultimately what adds excess weight to your body. It is almost impossible to avoid binge eating if you are continually burdening yourself with a backpack of guilt for your tendency to do what everyone else is *also* doing at this stage of human evolution, making mistakes and slipping up repeatedly. Where as tiny toddlers we learn by trial and error to walk, as adults we are doing much the same thing, frequently stumbling and falling and having to pick ourselves up and dust ourselves off as we navigate the challenges of life. The learning never stops! We're going to trip many times on our journey, and rather than beating up on ourselves for doing so, it is appropriate to show compassion and patience. If you want to live a life free of an obsession with food, *now* is the time to drop the heavy pack. You're human! Lighten up on yourself for the love of Pete!

Perhaps you can't see the miracle that you are because your focus is trained on what you don't like about yourself. If you are busy focusing on the flaws in a priceless diamond, you can't see its brilliance. While I absolutely agree that it is perfectly appropriate to observe yourself honestly and make efforts to correct your mistakes, focusing *exclusively* on what you perceive to be your imperfections is a one-way ticket to *depressionville*, where food becomes your Prozac.

Thinking that I was "bad" or not as good as others caused me to withhold love from myself for what I perceived as massive flaws. This punitive self-condemnation drove me to eat like a crazy woman. Alternatively, the more I was able to love myself (even my dark side), and forgive myself for my mistakes, the more I was able to let go of the anxiety and low self-esteem that was fueling my desires to overeat.

Awareness Opportunity

When I suggest that you too could love yourself more than you do today, how does it make you feel? What is the first thought that pops into your head when you think of the concept of "self-love"?

The reason I ask you to define self-love for *yourself* is because people all too frequently confuse it with self-absorption, selfishness and narcissism. When I was struggling with compulsive eating and low self-esteem, I would have been totally embarrassed to admit I loved myself. I would have thought that it would make me look conceited and haughty. It wasn't until I made the important distinction between self-love and an over-inflated ego that I could acknowledge my love for myself without any shame. So what's the difference?

Vanity, excessive self-promotion and self-absorption are *not* characteristics of self-love. Indeed they often point to the exact opposite, a lack of self-love (otherwise known as low self-esteem), which is being masked by overconfidence, superiority and narcissism. People who aren't aware of their own value often feel the need to brag about their achievements or possessions in order to gain respect or attention, and they typically have a limited ability to give to others. All their focus is instead directed toward themselves, trying to get their emotional needs met through various "highs" (attention from others, food, distractions, alcohol, power, possessions, drugs, sex, television, work) because their internal world feels so fragile, unsafe or even empty.

By contrast, people who love themselves have a healthy self-appreciation that does not preclude their caring deeply about others. In fact, it adds *enormously* to their ability to do so! They tend to be happy, healthy, centered, gracious, tolerant, courageous, humorous, giving, peaceful, non-judgmental, honest, self-respecting, abundant, forgiving, loving, appreciative, confident, humble, wise and gentle. Authentic self-love is the art and practice of honoring yourself, irrespective of what you look like or what you possess, and independent of what you have or have not yet achieved in your life. Self-love, when embodied, is accompanied by a deep sense of inner peace and contentment. You are consciously aware of your inherent value and you recognize the fact that you are a unique, magnificent and irreplaceable soul. Self-loving individuals create a safe inner sanctuary where they feel comfortable admitting to their dark side or "shadow qualities," which actually helps to reduce them.

The people I know who love themselves strike a healthy balance between confidence and humility. They love and appreciate who they are, but feel neither superior or inferior to anyone else, recognizing that as humans, we are all equals regardless of our life circumstances. They give and receive with equal pleasure. Their self-respect is reflected in their choices: they surround themselves with loving, supportive, healthy friends; they balance work, play and leisure time; and they take excellent care of their bodies. They stop themselves when they are tempted to judge because they recognize that judgment pollutes their own bodies as well as the planet. They take action to change the circumstances of their lives that are causing them consternation and surrender to events that are out of their control. As a result of all these self-loving behaviors, they are so happy and fulfilled that they give to others out of sheer gratitude. They understand their limitless power and capacity to manifest their deepest heart's desires so they are never envious of what other people possess. In fact, they care deeply and passionately about the well-being of others.

As you can see, far from being selfish, self-love is an incredibly healing and generous act, not just for yourself, but for anyone you come into contact with! It follows that the degree to which you honor and love yourself will dictate the extent to which you offer true unconditional love to others. I couldn't love at my fuller capacity until my relationship with myself was intact, prior to that point my love was still genuine, but it was also a more conditional love. And it didn't stop there. When I used to judge myself, I was far more likely to be critical of others. When I abused myself, I was more likely to mistreat others. When I neglected myself, I wasn't as present to my loved ones. When I was impatient with myself, I felt less tolerant of others. When I lied to myself, I was more prone to be dishonest with others. This is why practicing self-love is *the* most profound gift you can offer the world.

Self-love brings out the *best* of who you are, who we all are. It turns us into more loving friends, wives, husbands, sisters, brothers, mothers, fathers and leaders. The world is in desperate need of more individuals who truly love themselves and bring their most loving selves to their personal and professional lives as well as to leadership roles that influence the well-being of the planet. If you knew for a *fact* that loving yourself would make the world a better place, would it be easier for you to love yourself? If your answer was yes, then let the love affair begin.

Awareness Opportunity

The question of whether or not you love yourself, and just how much you love yourself, merits deep investigation because it will impact every experience in your life. The purpose of this next exercise is to help you determine whether or not you are in a truly loving relationship with yourself. Answering the following questions will offer you some additional insights and instigate some "aha" moments. Simply circle the ones that are a "yes" for you.

Do you compare yourself to other women?

Do you compare your body to other women's?

Are you uncomfortable spending time alone?

Do you look to others to approve of and validate you?

Are you unforgiving with yourself?

Do you feel ashamed of yourself because of what your body looks like?

Do you place more value upon what you look like rather than who you are inside?

Are you hard on yourself when you make a mistake?

Do you find it difficult to identify and express your feelings?

Are you afraid of your future because you doubt your abilities?

Do you worry about what others think of you?

Are you uncomfortable saying "no" when someone asks a favor?

Do you ignore your intuition, believing that others know better than you do?

Do you frequently feel unsure of yourself?

Do you fear criticism?

Do you feel like you don't "fit in"?

Do you repeatedly engage in behaviors that sabotage your own happiness?

Do you have a difficult time making your own needs a priority?

Do you accept unkind or inappropriate behavior from others?

Are you critical of yourself?

Do you use food to numb yourself to your feelings?

Do you deny yourself loving physical intimacy because you are embarrassed of your body?

Do you choose to be in relationships with people who do not support you?

Do you neglect your physical well-being?

Do you frequently get cranky and irritable with yourself and others?

Is it common for you to feel down or even depressed?

Do you have a need for perfection?

Do you feel responsible for others?

Do you feel nervous when something really good comes into your life?

Is it easier to take care of others than it is to take care of yourself?

All of these behaviors are little red flags that suggest you are not loving yourself to your full potential. If you circled "yes" to any, many or most of the questions, there is an opportunity to deepen your relationship with *you*, which is *fantastic* news, because when you better your relationship with yourself, *every single aspect of your life is positively impacted.* Let's go a little deeper.

Stand in front of a mirror and stare at your entire reflection for a few minutes. After this time is up, I invite you to spend the next two minutes looking directly into your own eyes. After you finish, please answer the following questions:

How did you *feel* as you looked at your reflection?

What were you *thinking* as you looked at yourself?

Were you judging yourself or appreciating yourself as you stared at your reflection?

If you had a difficult time looking at yourself, if you were drawn to judging yourself, if you feel anything less than respect and appreciation, it is a signal that you are somehow disconnected from the truth of your inherent value. If you generally feel unworthy, you are more likely to unintentionally sabotage yourself by making choices or repeating behaviors (e.g., compulsively eating) that impair your ability to enjoy life. If you are not aware of the innate beauty of your soul, you might also believe that unless your body matches the media-endorsed images adopted by our culture, you are not wonderful, attractive or desirable (ridiculous). You may also feel insecure around other people, as though they are "more than" or "better than" you (completely untrue).

Your own compulsion with food is letting you know that there are low-vibration ways you are thinking about yourself ("I'm not attractive. I'm not good enough.") or about your life ("I can't do that." "That will never happen for me." "Something bad might happen.") that are so upsetting to your state of mind that you are driven to eat. But do not despair, your discomfort and dissatisfaction with yourself or your life circumstances today will inspire you to go "within" to develop a heightened level of self-awareness and self-love.

<u>Yeah, But How Do I Do It?</u>

Here's more good news. There is *no* doubt that you have the ability to love yourself and your body and simultaneously overcome your addiction to food. At this point, however, you're probably thinking, "Okay, this sounds great, but how *exactly* do I set free this force for good? How, specifically, can I love myself more?" You see, love is both a feeling and a behavior. I am going to teach you a wide variety of ways to become more loving toward yourself, which, through practice, will also give you an increased *feeling* of self-love and all the goodies that come with it.

There are innumerable self-love practices, and I have placed them into two categories, one being mental self-love practices and the other physical. The mental side of self-love involves choosing *thoughts* and *beliefs* that honor and serve you and your body. The physical side involves choosing *behaviors* that serve you and your body. When you combine the two, big magic happens. Not the "saw the lady in half" type magic, but rather the miraculous and spiritual kind where you gain access to the profound joys and blissful experiences that make life worth living.

While the self-love practices are quite simple, they are not always easy...at first. We humans have a tendency to return to the well-worn path of our habits rather than venturing into the uncharted territory of new behaviors, which almost always requires more grit. When self-sabotaging patterns run deep, we often instinctively default to them out of habit. Like a muscle, however, the more you train and even push yourself to engage in loving behaviors, the stronger your new way of being will become. Self-love, although not always easy to attain, is eminently achievable through focus and, of course, the inevitable practice.

The Mental Game of Self-Love: Choose the Most Loving, Affirming and Healthy Thoughts You Can Conceive Of.

Awareness Opportunity

Take a moment to say each of the following statements aloud and allow yourself to feel the specific *feelings* that accompany each one. Stay with each statement for a few moments and tune into the place in your body where you feel the impact of your statement most obviously.

Statement #1: I am a kind, good hearted, lovely, divine individual who is capable of creating anything I want in my life. I love my body and am learning to take excellent care of it.

Statement #2: I feel unattractive and overweight, and I'll never lose these extra pounds because I can't control myself. I don't like how I look, and I don't know how to change that.

Now take a moment to write down the answers to the following questions:

How did statement #1 make you feel mentally?

How did it make you feel physically?

How did statement #2 make you feel mentally?

How about physically?

Chances are good that statement number one made you feel better than statement number two, simply because it is a "higher vibration" statement – a far more loving and inspiring perspective. On the second statement the vibrational bar is low; on the first, the bar is raised and the feeling it generates in your body will reflect that elevation. Raising the bar on your *thoughts* is the skill you want to master if you want to heal your relationship with yourself and your body. If you are looking to feel good, keep in mind that every thought generates a physical reaction!

Both positive and negative thoughts, when repeated enough times in your mind, become *beliefs*, and those beliefs then dictate your behaviors.

Thought Repeated = Belief = Dictates Behavior

A low-vibration thought ("I'll never lose this weight") repeated in your highly impressionable mind *consistently* becomes a negative belief, which drives the negative behavior of overeating.

Higher vibration thinking *always* leads to higher vibration results in the long term. Thinking highly of yourself, thinking optimistically about your circumstances and focusing on solutions to your challenges will lead you to the best choices available. This is in part because the way you choose to perceive any situation can, and will, dictate your feelings around it, which will then influence your choices and actions. To think "high," you've got to crowd out the negative conversation running through your mind with a more positive one. This practice is the *golden ticket* to deeper levels of joy. Erasing the old internal conversation by replacing it with a positive one is tantamount to changing the way you will experience life.

When I am trying to replace a negative line of thinking with a positive one so I can *feel* better, I'll ask myself, "What is the most positive perspective, the highest thoughts I can have on my circumstances in this moment?" Then I dig around in my mind and heart until I find it. How do I know when I've found it? I feel better *instantly*. I can't tell you how many times I've calmed myself down and reversed my mood with this practice. Without exaggerating, it is completely life altering. I have also found that it helps dramatically to speak the more positive perspective *out loud* in order to drown out the negative thoughts that can get quite boisterous. When my thoughts are *really* dragging me down I dialogue with myself the way I would with a good friend, patiently and supportively. I now know that my low-vibration thoughts often show up habitually and that positive thinking is a practice.

Do you want to *feel* better on a daily basis? Then you have to *think* better on a daily basis. It is that simple. I'm not talking about merely repeating positive affirmations; I'm talking about upgrading your overall thinking process. The more negative your thinking, the more you will feel depressed, insecure and fearful. The more loving your thoughts, the more you will know internal peace. And by loving I mean not just *kind* thoughts, but wise, centered and life-enhancing perspectives that encourage you to know how capable you are as you look for the optimum solution in every single situation you face.

If you regularly engage in this mental practice, you will, without question, experience greater levels of happiness. This is not just because your thoughts are making you feel more joyous, but also because high-vibration (positive and healthy) thoughts lead to high-vibration outcomes, whether that outcome is releasing excess weight, finding a career you love, attracting a wonderful partner or just having a wonderful day. When your thoughts about yourself are respectful and appreciative, you will begin to attract more positive experiences of all kinds into your life. It will be easier to achieve any goals you set for yourself, whether they are personal, professional, financial or, in the case of achieving your natural weight, physical.

I'm not going to pretend like this practice is a walk in the park when you first begin. As you likely already know, it's much harder to think high-vibration thoughts than it sounds. Frankly, it ain't always easy to look for the grander perspective, the more loving approach and the gift and ultimate solution in every situation–especially when things are not flowing smoothly, or someone hurts your feelings or you are not getting *what* you want *when* you want it. But if you want to improve your overall mood and start having more peak moments, you have to buck up and do it anyway because there's no faster way to joy than retraining your brain. You know the high you get when you get really good at something? Well multiply that yummy feeling by ten or twenty or even a hundred, because that's how phenomenal it feels to use your mind to think "high and healthy." You have to dig into your intestinal fortitude to make this happen, to be strong, to cowboy or cowgirl up even when the going gets tough.

Repeatedly choose those thoughts that are kind to yourself, inspiring, calming and *smart*. A smart thought is one that empowers you and brings you to a more peaceful place (and here's the important part), *regardless of your circumstances*. For example, if I am feeling angry with myself because after a weekend of bingeing I can't fit into my favorite skirt, I can deal with it in a number of ways. My prior knee-jerk response, before I knew the powerful influence of my thoughts on my level of personal empowerment (or lack thereof), would have been a punishing thought such as "Ugh, I'm so mad at myself. Now I look horrible in this skirt, it's way too tight. Get a hold of your eating, you little weakling. What is wrong with you! You are never going to lose weight." I'd attack myself savagely and then slink off into my day, depressed and ashamed. This negative inner diatribe would *always* make me feel much worse about my situation, which would propel me to head, usually in a zombie-like state, right for the pantry.

I finally realized that when I am mean, to myself and my body, I eat a lot more!

My new and improved response means cutting myself a break when I can't fit into my skirt and accessing a gentle voice of compassion for myself. My experience has shown me that a loving, encouraging voice is a far stronger force for personal growth than a punishing one, which is why I have far fewer impulses to binge. My inner dialogue today would sound more like this: "I can understand why you would feel upset about not fitting into your pink skirt, but being mad at yourself will only make you feel worse. Your only job today is to be gentle with yourself and that will calm you so you don't feel the need for that box of Twinkies. The smartest thing you can do is to be good to yourself today." If I'm alone, I kindly coach myself out loud so that I get the message loud and clear.

I have figured out that it is a *much* wiser choice to think higher if I want to calm myself, accurately assess my options given my circumstances and make the kind of choices that lead to the best turnout. Remember to think *high* to calm *down*. When you are in a truly peaceful place, you are simply not interested in eating unless you are hungry.

This practice of choosing my thoughts wisely required me to first slow down and observe my thoughts in order to assess and explore their quality. It was extremely important for me to become aware of the nature of my thinking on a daily basis because my negative thoughts were always producing negative moods and consequently negative outcomes. When you begin to observe or "witness" your thoughts, you will also begin to notice with greater accuracy and consistency if they are self-defeating (negative/low- vibration) or self-empowering (positive/high-vibration). Practicing high-vibration thinking, even when I didn't feel like it, helped to reduce my anxiety and depression and increase my happiness, my euphoria factor.

Remember, sometimes it takes a little time to shift to a higher way of thinking. Nineteenth century author and philosopher Henry David Thoreau said, "As a single footstep will not make a path on the earth so a single thought will not make a pathway in the mind. To make a deep *physical* path, we walk again and again. To make a deep *mental* path we must think over and over the kind of thoughts we wish to dominate our lives." Your resolute and committed *focus* on the life-affirming practice of thinking "high" will bring you the "high" feelings you are reaching for in food. By deliberately keeping your mind focused on the healthiest *thoughts*, you will be one giant step closer to achieve your healthiest *weight*!

Awareness Opportunity

Here is an opportunity to gain a deeper understanding of the *nature* of your mind, to familiarize yourself with its character. In order to do this you are going to take a stab at meditation. Don't worry, it won't hurt or bore you to death, at worst it may make you uncomfortable. I invite you to put this book down and for the next three to five minutes (or more if you are inspired) focus *only* on your breath. Try not to think of anything else but your breath flowing in and out. If a thought pops into your head, merely acknowledge it ("Ah, look, I'm thinking about what I'm going to make for dinner."). Then return your focus to your breathing. A great way to maintain your focus is to let your breath be louder than your thoughts. Gently exaggerate your breath if your thoughts are sneaking in. After you are finished, please answer the following questions:

What was your experience with meditation?

Did you notice that there was a constant flow of thoughts going through your head?

Did you find that keeping your attention on your breath was challenging?

How did your thoughts make you feel?

As you can see, trying to divert your attention from your thoughts can feel like attempting to stop a fully loaded freight train dead in its tracks when it's heading down a steep grade. This is the nature of the mind. It is compulsively and relentlessly active. I compare it to a wild horse that you can't saddle up and ride easily. Or in some cases, it's a bucking bronco that jerks you around mentally until you attempt to seek relief in the form of a treat.

Here's why meditation is so important: It can help you to practice the art of *silencing* your thoughts or help you to get to the space *between* thoughts. It supports you in recognizing and knowing how to *stop* those negative thoughts before they drive you to overeat. If the goal of meditation is to *silence* your thoughts, the goal of *witnessing* your thoughts is to support you in raising their vibration. Both are superb mental trainings.

When I started to observe my own thoughts, whether it was when I was trying to meditate or just engaged in my day-to-day activities, I couldn't *believe* how many of them were low-vibration! Even with my eating issues, I considered myself a pretty positive person, but when I *really* started watching my stream of consciousness, I discovered a line of negative and fearful thinking that surprised me. I had lots of "worried" thoughts about the future and all too frequently indulged in self-denigrating thoughts. I had to pay close attention and start catching myself in the act of low-vibration thinking to bring a halt to it. By being aware of your thoughts, watching and not judging, you too will start to catch yourself in the act of the compulsive negative thinking that fuels compulsive eating.

Do you have an idea of how many thoughts you think a day? Take a rough guess. Research shows that humans think an average of 60,000 thoughts a day and of these 60,000 thoughts, *ninety percent* of them are the same ones we had yesterday, and the day before and the day before! And studies show that 77% of these thoughts run towards the negative, some variation on the theme "I'm not good enough," or worries about the future, regrets about the past or judgments of others. Our brains, in part because we are living in patterns and routines (waking up at the same time, going to work, coming home, spending time with the same people), are unconsciously trained to revert to the same exact thoughts we had before ("I've got so much to do." "I ate too much." "I am not doing enough."). And if most of our thoughts fall into the "fear of the future" or "I'm not good enough" category, it is not at all surprising that many of us are bummed out, depressed victims of our untamed minds which prattle on relentlessly. "I can't do anything right." "I'll never be thin." "I can't control my appetite." "Something might go wrong." "What if something bad happens to me?" "My life is boring." "I can't do it." "I'm miserable." "I don't have enough time." "I have too much to do." "She has a better body than I do." Oy! With each negative thought, you are repeatedly self-administering tiny doses of depression fuel. If you said *out loud* all the fearful or self-deprecating thoughts that dance through your mind all day, you'd be far more tapped into your detrimental thinking habits.

Low-vibration thinking is a pervasive human condition. We are *all* falling prey to it collectively, but we usually don't notice that we're doing it because everyone else is doing it too. Redirecting your thinking patterns is one of the most powerful practices for personal happiness and growth. It is one of, if not the greatest "secrets" to living in joy. All you have to do is begin, today, to "watch" your thoughts and observe your stream of consciousness. When you catch yourself thinking low-vibration, rejecting a body part, or any part of who you are (e.g., "I hate my stomach." "I'm not as pretty as she is." "I can't do this."), replace the low-vibration thought as quickly as you can with a high-vibration one.

You can direct your thoughts as surely as you can direct your body. You can tell your body to sit down, break into a sprint or lie down and it will do as you order. Likewise you can tell your mind to "stop" or to "be quiet" as you access your heart and the high-vibration thoughts that will lift your mood and inspire you to make healthier choices in all areas of your life. It is all under your command. You are the director of the dialogue in your mind, so focus on supervising and guiding it consciously and confidently.

In order to silence the negative thoughts you are having about yourself, I suggest acknowledging something wonderful about yourself: "I'm a really kind person." "I have the ability to manifest anything I want in my life." "I deserve to be happy." "When I am good to myself, I make the world a better place." There is no end to the wonderful things about you. Be fierce and unrelenting in your quest to focus on *those* aspects of who you are. See each and every negative thought as an obstacle to your happiness and disintegrate it with a high-vibration thought.

When you find yourself projecting into the future and feeling fearful of what might happen, what can you do? Redirect your thoughts in the most gentle, affectionate and affirming direction possible. For example, if you are thinking, "I'm scared that I will never lose this weight," override that thought with one like "Of course I will reach my natural weight, and by loving myself I'll get there even faster." Be your own rooting section, your own enthusiastic cheerleader, your own private dedicated and inspirational coach instead of your harshest critic.

Any time you find yourself thinking in a self-defeating way, gently guide your mind toward healthy thoughts and perspectives like a loving friend would. Just like you would choose a ripe, juicy peach over a bruised, moldy one, choose your thoughts selectively. Don't allow your mind to rule your world. Use your mind instead to *change* your mood and to make your life a much sweeter dream. Your high-vibration thoughts come from a heart-centered space. There is a nurturing and loving voice deep down inside you–inside all of us, that is much easier to hear when you breathe deeply, *really* deeply, and place your hand on your heart.

If you are having a difficult time accessing that gentle voice for yourself, think of a person or an animal you love unconditionally and the tone of voice you would use with them. It may take a while to trust that kinder voice. But with time you will see it is *always* available to you when you listen for it. With continual practice, it will eventually be the loudest and most dominant one in your head. That sweet internal voice makes it safer and easier to investigate your feelings to determine what fears, worries and self-doubts are driving your hunger urges. I think of the "sweet" voice as one that an especially loving, kind, adoring, patient and wise mother would use with her children.

A loving *internal* dialogue makes your *external* life flow smoothly, and opens you to the joys of life that are always there for you. It creates a sacred inner space for you to turn to in times of crisis or confusion. It is the voice that encourages you to wait to eat the piece of chocolate cake until you are hungry rather than trying to persuade you to eat it now even though your body is telling you "no thanks." Your internal nurturing maternal voice will be the gentle one that, in combination with your firm paternal voice, will set the limits for your child-like side that wants the Oompa Loompa now!

Awareness Opportunity

Write down a thought(s) you frequently have about yourself that you consider low-vibration.

Now write a high-vibration thought(s) you can defer to the next time you catch yourself thinking in a self-sabotaging way.

The Tamed vs. the Untamed Mind

Here's an important distinction that can help you to differentiate your low- vibration thoughts from your high ones in the most effective fashion. Think of your mind as having two parts, one part "tamed," the other "untamed." Low-vibration thoughts are always generated by your "untamed mind" and will always make you feel some variation of "bad." Your untamed mind has also been referred to as the "ego" mind, the "monkey" mind and the "primitive" mind.

It is the irrational and fearful part of your mind that is constantly critical of you, repeatedly takes you out of the present moment, fuels worries about the future and often keeps you unwisely focused on regrets about the past. It fills you with self-doubt and uncertainty. Your untamed mind is an overly dramatic, insatiable, demanding, sneaky, negative troublemaker. It is the part of your mind that is critical, judgmental and perpetually in anxiety of some kind. It also keeps you relentlessly focused on what you *don't* want rather than what you *do* want. Your untamed mind generates the ugly thoughts that rob you of your wallet in the moment and your life savings in the long term. Most of us spend the majority of our time in our untamed mind (remember that ninety percent statistic?). We are victims of a part of our mind we don't even realize we have! No *wonder* so many of us are turning to mood-enhancing medications!

Even if we *are* aware that most of our thoughts are worry-driven or negative, most of us don't know that we have control over them. We are unaware that we can silence the untamed mind by redirecting it toward higher vibration thoughts. I *always* know that my untamed mind is the culprit if I am feeling bad, depressed, insecure or worried. I also now know (thank heavens) that I can transform my thoughts and my mood if I choose to think high-vibration.

64

In contrast to your untamed mind, you also have what I refer to as a "tamed" mind, also called the conscious mind. It's the part of your mind that contains memories, facts and figures. It is your "intelligent" mind, which helps you to solve problems, find solutions to personal challenges, organize your thoughts and prioritize. Your tamed mind is of great benefit to you, helping you to make good choices and practice discernment. It is also the part of your mind that can help you to focus on what you *want*, rather than what you *don't* want, which will help you to manifest your desires and dreams much faster. The sweet and nurturing voice you turn on yourself helps you to access the wisdom of the tamed mind more readily. Breathing consciously, with long, drawn-out inhales and exhales, also helps tremendously.

How do you know when your untamed mind is engaged? Through your *feelings*. If you feel anxious, frightened, tense, sad, depressed, fearful, frustrated or uncomfortable, there is a high probability that you are in the grips of your untamed mind. Your untamed mind will either ride you too hard, take you out of the present moment by worrying about what might or might not happen in the future, make you regret a past choice or resist a circumstance in your life over which you have no control. The untamed mind is like having a full-time worry wart/nag/pessimist in your head. It is paranoid, irrational and misleading. It is clever because it gets you to believe its delusions, but it is not intelligent because it gives really bad advice. It comes across as though it knows a lot, luring you into a line of thinking that will wear you down, but it is actually quite ignorant. If you are not aware that your untamed mind has taken over, it can continue to prevent you from enjoying the moment in the short term and your life in the long term. I can limit my true potential and even wreck a significant portion of my life if I'm not careful to watch my mind and master it.

Becoming aware of the nature of your mind is the first step towards learning how to get it to work *for* you rather than against *you*. It is *also* the key to averting binge eating. To put it in a nutshell, the better you think, the better you feel and the less you want to overeat. If you want to get to the root of an uncomfortable feeling, if you want to figure out exactly *why* you are feeling bad, take a moment to stop, breathe deeply, put your hand on your heart and reflect on the thoughts you had that preceded the feeling. This will allow you to identify and correct the untamed thought that got you riled up. Were you judging your body? Were you worrying what others were thinking about you? If you have slid into "I'm not good enough" or "I'm not doing enough" mode, this usually translates into thoughts like "I'm not getting enough accomplished," "I am not doing it right," "I don't look attractive," "I don't fit in." Staying "tuned in" to your feelings will help you to recognize when you are cracking the whip on yourself or indulging in depleting thoughts. The uncomfortable feelings will *always* pass, without question. Allow yourself, with the assistance of deep breathing, to temporarily sink into the intense feeling, like you would an extra-hot bath, and watch the discomfort drain away once you adjust to the heat.

Do you ever remember as a child thinking that you saw something scary in a dark room, something that, once you turned the lights on, you realized was not there? It is the same with your fears and worries about the future. They need the light of your understanding and focus in order to expose their illusory nature. Fear is predominantly a free-floating, random response to the voice of your untamed mind, which you must simply redirect and reassure in order to turn its volume down.

Watch Your Mind in Action

As you did with your negative thoughts about *yourself*, just begin to take note of your *worried and fearful* thoughts. You don't have to like them, but don't fight the feelings or let them intimidate you. Resistance only makes them stronger! Simply observe them, and search your memory to see what low-vibration thought stimulated the fear. Then tune into the place in your body where you feel fearful. Oftentimes fear shows up in the chest area, stomach or the throat. Once you have identified *where* it resides, place your hands on that body part, breathe deeply and gently remind yourself that even though your fears *feel* real, the overwhelming majority of the time, they are not. I used to worry *all* the time that something big and bad might happen to me or someone I loved. Whether it was an earthquake or a life-threatening illness, my untamed mind would run wild with random thoughts about what "could" happen. These thoughts would pop up out of the blue and I could make myself quite miserable by indulging them. Now I know they are misguided tricks of my untamed mind and I know to remind myself that there is no reason to worry. I'll sometimes say "no," forcefully and out loud to the part of my untamed mind that stirs up trouble, and sometimes my fears disappear instantaneously.

If you take the time to calm and center yourself and observe your inner dialogue, you will be able to more accurately assess whether your worries are inflated creations of your untamed mind or whether they represent legitimate concerns that you need to address (e.g., overdue bills, an uncomfortable conversation, a health concern).

Instead of reaching for something to eat when you feel frightened or worried, now is the time to figure out what you *really* need. Sometimes it's a big hug from someone you love, other times it is simply digging into a project you have been avoiding. Most of the time, the only thing you need is to shift to high-vibration thinking, to purposefully reach for the thought that makes you feel good, or great, or at least better than the fear- driven or judgmental one that got you eating compulsively.

This is not about being oblivious to negative conditions in your life; rather, thinking "high" or "higher" is merely the smartest way to give yourself the physical and mental energy to deal with your circumstances. It can help you shut down the untamed mind so that you can focus on *solutions* rather than the problem, to focus on what you *do* have rather than what you do not, to identify your opportunity in every situation so that you can move ahead in your life rather than staying a victim of your circumstances.

As you progress in the practice of watching your thoughts, over time you will get more familiar with and savvy to the shenanigans of your untamed mind. Remember to let your uncomfortable feelings alert you to the fact that your untamed mind is dominating your state of mind. Even the simple feat of catching your untamed mind in the act will give you easier access to your tamed mind. Your tamed mind will remind you to think high, to reach for the grander perspective, to embrace yourself fully by acknowledging yourself in some way. It will suggest that rather than judging someone else harshly, your thoughts should be compassionate and understanding. Your tamed mind will also lead you away from illusory worries about the future by reminding you that you have the ability to handle whatever comes your way. Obviously, your tamed mind is far wiser and cooler than your untamed mind and it is easier to access when you stop to acknowledge your uncomfortable feelings.

Mastering Your Mood

When I am feeling *really* overwhelmed, I keep my untamed mind in check in a number of powerful ways. One is gratitude. This is the most powerful tool at my disposal to change my mood and my mind. I start by acknowledging all the gifts I have been blessed with, the things I love about my life, both the little and the big, and I focus my attention on the excitement I have for all the great moments I am certain are coming in the future. I search for the highest perspective on whatever situation I am facing in order to calm my panicked, untamed mind.

When that's not working and I'm *still* feeling overwhelmed, I use another tactic. I turn my thoughts towards those who are struggling with something even *more* challenging than what I am facing. I have only to pick up the newspaper or turn on the news to hear about the hardships of other people around the world to put my own worries and complaints into proper perspective. I remind myself, "Gee, I could be living in a war-torn country living in constant fear for my life" or "I could be living in a place where I have to walk for two days just to get clean water." These thoughts are stark reality checks that propel me to view my circumstances from a more centered place. After thinking of others who are enduring *extreme* hardship, suddenly anything I am facing seems *imminently* more manageable. I'm not suggesting that you ignore or downplay your own personal challenges. I am always understanding and gentle with myself as I navigate my own. But I have found it's *much* easier to deal with my circumstances when I'm not overwhelmed by my untamed mind, which is whipping me into a frenzy by attempting to convince me that I have a *really* big problem on my hands when something didn't go the way I had planned, or I'm put on "hold" longer than I'd like or when I don't like the number I see on the scale.

I realize that my problems are "champagne" problems compared to many others and I am humbled by this truth. Sometimes, *especially* when I'm tired, or overly busy and overworked, I will have to use both tactics to "double-team" my untamed mind so I don't end up stress eating. I'll usually *start* with gratitude and then use my compassionate thoughts for those who have it much harder as a reality check that allows me to navigate my own challenges with far more grace. From this "grace place" I can choose my thoughts around whatever I am facing in a far more sensible and empowered fashion.

The great poet and philosopher Ralph Waldo Emerson once said, "Man is what he thinks all day long." Define for yourself how *you* want to think, with the understanding that it will determine your destiny. And practice mastering your mind and thoughts, daily! From this place, your life experience will shift towards a far higher degree of fulfillment and happiness and simultaneously allow you to achieve your goals as they relate not *only* to your body, but also to your life circumstances in general–your career, your relationships, your hopes and dreams. If you are not convinced, try it for one week, or even a day, heck, try it for an hour and you'll get to see firsthand the incredible difference your high-vibration thinking makes to your ability to live your day to its fullest!

Below are the specific steps to raise the bar on your thoughts so you can center yourself and move beyond an urge to binge:

1. Become aware of your uncomfortable feeling(s).

2. Identify the place in your body where the discomfort is being held and put your hand on that spot.

3. Breathe deeply into that place.

4. Pinpoint the thought(s) you had that drove the urge to eat.

5. Raise the vibration of that thought to a higher frequency by directing your thoughts in the most loving, affirming, solution-oriented direction available to you. Coach yourself in a kind and gentle manner. (Think of the person you love the most and use the same tone of voice in which you would speak to them if you knew they were troubled.)

6. From that safe and loving place, determine what you truly need (e.g., to be heard and acknowledged by a friend, a gentle reminder that it is all going to be okay, a gentle nudge to take action on a circumstance that is renting space in your head) and give it to yourself instead of resorting to food.

Now that you have a better understanding of the *mental* side of practicing self-love, it is time to move on to the highly pleasurable (most of the time) physical side.

The Physical Game: Engage in Self-Loving Activities Every Chance You Get

In my early twenties I fell into a serious life rut. I had a job as a manager of a cosmetics department at Emporium Capwell in San Francisco and I was in charge of more than thirty employees. I wasn't the *least* bit motivated by my work, very few things about it were fulfilling and enjoyable, but it was considered a good job for someone in her early twenties, and I just stuck with it out of familiarity and lethargy. During this chapter of my life, television was often my evening companion. I'd sit, night after night, channel surfing and sifting through the contents of my refrigerator for my next snack. I'd graze from one flavor to the next, from sweet foods to salty ones, from hot dishes to cold ones. I'd go to sleep late at night and I'd wake in the morning with a food hangover and numbly head back into work. In short, I didn't have a life I was excited about. I was just getting by. I was unfulfilled personally and professionally, but I didn't know how, or was too afraid to initiate big changes in my life. I couldn't define my passions because I wasn't slowing down long enough to get in touch with them. I was always trying to fill myself with something sugary because there were not enough sweet moments in my life.

Part of the reason so many of us are not as happy as we could be is because we are living a lifestyle that doesn't bring us very much pleasure. We are frequently working jobs we are not passionate about, involved in relationships that fall short of our dreams and struggling daily to create balance in our lives. In today's hyper-fast multitasking society, we are pretty adept at getting things done, but not nearly as consistent when it comes to having fun or engaging in pastimes we absolutely love. Being happy and fulfilled requires choosing and creating a lifestyle you are passionate about, one that makes you excited to get out of bed in the morning. In hindsight I can see that many of my emotional appetites were related to the fact that I wanted more excitement, fun, fulfillment, purpose, passion and adventure in my life. Most of the time I was surviving rather than thriving, so food became my consolation prize. Once I began to break away from my old entrenched ways of being, to push myself outside my comfort zones, my life began to be far more enticing and my appetites calmed down.

If you knew that you had only ten years to live, or even two, would you be spending your time differently than you are today? Would you be treating yourself differently? Making braver choices that make you feel more fully alive? Being more selective about *what* you do and *whom* you do it with? If you don't take time to contemplate what *exactly* would make you feel loved and joyful, you can't start taking action to create it. If there is no destination, there's little reason to move forward. Defining and creating a life you are joyous about is a *tremendous* act of self-love. Living in a setting or home environment that delights your senses and makes you feel safe and peaceful, surrounding yourself and spending time with loving friends, taking care of your body, having a career you enjoy, actively participating in your passions—these are all goals to work towards in order to show *yourself* that you are devoted to your own happiness.

Staying in a routine that is unfulfilling is an indication, a red flag, that you are not making yourself enough of a priority. To experience life at its fullest, you must make your own happiness one of your top goals. There are an *infinite* number of self-loving behaviors and only you can know for sure what nurturing behaviors positively impact your life and need to be engaged in with constancy. Take a moment and read a "starter" list of self-loving behaviors.

<u>Self-Loving Acts</u>:

Getting enough sleep

Meditating

Paying yourself a compliment

Getting a massage

Saying "no" when you feel overwhelmed

Forgiving yourself when you make an error in judgment

Making your feelings equally as important as anyone else's

Balancing work and play (i.e., some time for fun planned into every day)

Going dancing

Sleeping in

Spending time with family

Playing a musical instrument

Treating yourself to something beautiful

Having a meal prepared for you

Spending time with close friends

Having someone help you with your housework

Designing a retirement plan

Getting a manicure/pedicure

Taking a leisurely walk in Mother Nature

Taking yoga classes

Wearing comfortable clothes

Being patient with yourself

Cooking yourself a healthy meal

Having health insurance

Gardening

Dancing around your house

Playing a competitive sport

Doing volunteer work

Working out

Getting rid of excess possessions

Limiting your television time

Coaching yourself (i.e., having a loving internal dialogue)

Slowing down or stopping to nurture yourself when you are upset

Having an organized home/workspace

Being able to say "no" without feeling guilty

Buying yourself a piece of clothing that makes you feel beautiful

Reading inspirational books

Getting a supportive coach/counselor

Taking care of your skin

Stretching

Seeing an inspirational movie

Planning a day where you have no obligations or commitments

Driving someplace beautiful

Limiting your exposure to "negative" influences (e.g., violent television, films)

Spending time with animals

Having a good cry

Singing

Having fresh flowers in your home

Going to the beach

Taking a nap when you are tired

Getting dressed up

Hiking

Limiting communication with unsupportive family/friends

Taking a long, hot bath

Sitting down and doing absolutely nothing

Spending time alone

Working on a creative project (e.g., painting, sculpting, interior decorating)

Writing (poetry, music, stories)

Baking

Drinking water

Eating healthy food

Learning something new

Riding a bike

Asking for support

Taking a long, hot shower

Swimming

Simplifying your life

Going to the country

Nature watching (birds, flowers, wildlife)

Listening to music

Lighting a candle

Praying

Forgiving yourself when you make a mistake

Doing volunteer work

Working in balance

Being around children

Setting a boundary with someone who is behaving unfairly or unkindly

Taking breaks several times a day to rejuvenate

Other self-loving activities:

Awareness Opportunity

Write down in a journal the ten activities (plus any you thought of on your own) that would make you feel joyful and loved if you did them for yourself on a regular basis.

And now don't think about it, but, as they say, just do it! Even if you don't feel motivated, push yourself past your resistance. Call upon your inner champion (don't worry, you have one, we all do!) to give you that extra nudge. Prioritize your choices in a way that brings balance and harmony into your everyday life. Each day should be as close a representation as possible to the overall snapshot of your life. For the self-loving individual, every day includes not just productivity, but creativity, fun, physicality and some form of connection with their spiritual side. There *is* time for it all, even though your untamed mind may try to convince you that there is not. Craft your life like you would a movie with you as the director. Again, *you* are in charge–no one else can do it for you.

Engaging regularly in activities you know are good for you, mentally and physically, is tantamount to being self-loving. If you are not engaging in the things that bring you the greatest levels of peace and joy regularly, it is difficult to experience even a small percentage of the pleasure that is available to you. Most of us would be horrified to think that we neglected a baby or a child's needs, but we *do* neglect our own needs repeatedly without thinking twice about it and then experience the negative side effects that accompany not making ourselves a priority.

In the case of compulsive overeaters, we often substitute food for self-loving activities: a candy bar for a nap, a piece of pizza instead of a ten-minute walk in the park, a bowl of pasta instead of snuggling into a cozy chair with a good book. The more self-loving activities you incorporate into your life, the less you will have to turn to food to make yourself feel better. You will *already* be "feeling better" if you are repeatedly engaging in self-loving choices, and it feels *wonderful* to be living a life that is filled with exciting adventures and unique experiences!

Happily, I have found that the better I treat myself, the better life treats me! The surprising thing was that even when I started treating myself a *little* bit better, my life got a *lot* better. A foundation of self-love provided me with a feeling of inner serenity that serves as a solid anchor throughout any stormy seas that show up in my life. I now expect that the Divine is on my team, and that like a loving parent, it wants me to be filled with joy and peace, realizing that when I am in those states, I can offer the best of myself to this world.

I understand that it can sometimes be difficult to give yourself the love that you easily give to others. I recommend starting with small self-loving behaviors to get you warmed up for the big show. Something as simple as apologizing to yourself when you come down hard on yourself for making a mistake can make a big difference over time. Loving and respecting yourself is a prerequisite for a happy life. You deserve to have everything your heart desires; every human being on the planet does and you are no exception.

We all want to feel good. And, we are designed, genetically, to desire and seek out all the goodness in life, which is why we have little patience for the experiences that are unpleasant. Nobody really likes to feel bad! It's part of the reason compulsive overeating has become so rampant. So, if your only anti-pain coping skill is food, it is not surprising you would resort to it constantly. Which is *precisely* why you must have other satisfying and nurturing activities to supplement the eating habit!

Keep a list somewhere in your kitchen of the activities that nurture and fulfill you, perhaps posted in your pantry or on your refrigerator (or both). Read it first thing every morning. Purposefully engage in one of the activities before turning to a snack you are truly not hungry for. If you can breathe through or transcend the urge to eat just once a day and turn to a self-loving activity instead, you will, over time, build your capacity to overcome *all* non-hunger related urges to eat. You will be flexing your muscle of willpower and gradually losing desire to compulsively overeat. You've *got* to be bold, strong and focused to make this happen. You've got to bring out that self-loving inner warrior and muscle up.

As additional incentive, keep in mind that being self-loving is an act of great benefit to the world. Each time you engage in a self-loving activity, know that you are making the world a kinder and better place through your action. Think of it as a form of service each time you are compassionate with yourself, each time you slow down and nurture yourself with an activity that makes your heart sing. If each of us engaged in self-loving practices regularly, the world would be delightfully transformed for the better. Be a part of the "self-love movement" and do your bit to reverse the impact of living in a world where we often forget to love the person we will be spending the rest of our lives with—ourselves.

*****

"If anything is sacred, the human body is sacred."

—Walt Whitman

Chapter 3

Love Your Body

How Loving the Body You Have Can Help You Achieve Your Natural Weight

The human body is a miracle of nature, so advanced, so astoundingly *brilliant* and complex that even the most intelligent, well-educated and well-respected scientists in the world cannot explain some of its functions. Without question, your body holds a genius that is incomparable to *any* other known entity. Even a single cell in your body is an incredible marvel, possessing enough data to fill one thousand 600-page books. And that's in just *one* cell, which measures a mere 1/1000th of a centimeter! It has been estimated that your body has over one hundred trillion of these microscopic libraries of information.

Your body is a fantastic phenomenon, a creative, imaginative and adaptable system designed to support your survival in the harshest of conditions. It has an intelligence that the most technologically superior computers on the planet cannot come *close* to competing with. And as if that's not enough (what more could we ask for?), it is also set up to provide you with *unlimited* sensory delights (oh, that!). Our bodies give us entrée to an infinite number of physical and emotional pleasures every single day; visual pleasures such as the sight of an explosive rainbow, a deluxe sunset on a warm tropical beach, oral pleasures such as the taste of a creamy dessert, tactile pleasures such as the joy of a hug from a sweet child, or a romantic kiss, auditory pleasures such as listening to music that makes your heart sing along, olfactory delights such as the scent of warm cinnamon bread baking when you enter a toasty kitchen, sensual pleasures such as a massage that lasts for hours, and entire body pleasures such as those affiliated with the excitement of attaining a long sought after goal or even the rushes of euphoria that typify falling deeply in love. Your body is a sacred temple, an unfathomably wonderful gift, a generous blessing. Lucky for you, it is your insightful and devoted companion throughout your life.

Given that it houses our hearts and souls, the human body is the most precious life form on this planet. (Can you bring to mind anything that you possess that even comes close?) However, in spite of being an indisputable treasure, the human body is tragically under-appreciated, neglected and abused. If each of us *really* understood what we possess, if we were really able to grasp just how much of a miracle our bodies are, we would be awestruck in humble appreciation of our good fortune. Rather than whining about what we perceive as its deficiencies and flaws, we would absolutely accept and care for it with respect and appreciation, *exactly* as it is today, irrespective of its shape or weight. Instead, most of us judge our bodies as though they were our worst enemy. This is a heartbreaking reality, because our judgments of our bodies are, in very large part, responsible for the obesity epidemic we are experiencing worldwide.

The fact is that it is *very* hard to feel motivated to take care of something you don't care about. Conversely, when you care deeply for and truly honor your body, you will be far more likely to make the healthiest choices for it. It is the *caring* that creates the connection, which drives the healthy behaviors. When I started to honor my body, I found that I was far more likely to eat nutritious foods, exercise regularly, get plenty of rest and pamper it. When I didn't appreciate it, well...you know the story. I would repeatedly make unhealthy and shortsighted choices that would sabotage my desire to release my excess weight.

I physically cringe when I think back on the years during which I neglected and abused my body. It makes me sad to think I was so bad to something that was so good to me. It is a little like looking back on the sweet boyfriend you took for granted when you were too young and immature to see how giving, loyal and loving he was. I was so busy looking at what my body *wasn't* that I couldn't see what it was, and I deeply regret how I treated it. I was outright "rude" to my body: I neglected it, said mean things to it and ignored it repeatedly.

This behavior disconnected me from my body. It severed my ability to hear it and receive its wisdom and gifts of pleasure on many levels. I literally cut the lines of communication as I overate uncontrollably. I stuffed my helpless body with food even when it protested, and then I was mad at it for being bigger than I wanted it to be. I couldn't hear it telling me to stop eating because I was unwilling to listen to it. I ignored it when it told me to get to bed through obvious feelings of exhaustion and instead changed the channel and whipped up another snack. I shut out its signals for satiation as I served myself an additional portion. Like putting a gag on a wise guru, I stifled its communications. Why?

Because at the time it felt too overwhelming to deal with the intense feelings it was communicating. Like millions of other men and women, I had found that the fastest and most dependable way to get me "out of my body," where all the discomfort was taking place, was by numbing myself with food. Obviously, there were substantial consequences to this pattern because when I was disconnected from my body, I was *far* more prone to engage in *other* unhealthy behaviors that contributed to my weight spiraling up, and up, and up.

During that period of my life I rarely got enough sleep, choosing instead to watch television until the wee hours of the morning. I ate predominantly low nutrient, high- sugar foods and ignored my body's cravings for fresh, whole foods. I resisted exercise, either because I was too embarrassed to do it in public or because I didn't want to feel uncomfortable or bored. I rarely drank water, which is part of the reason I would hit a wall in the middle of the day and used sugar or caffeine to jack my system up when I was tired. I purged after huge meals, used laxatives when I felt bloated and took appetite suppressants to curb my hunger. I also spent most of my time indoors, rarely getting fresh air as I either watched a large amount of television (i.e., watched other people doing interesting things rather than doing them myself) or spent hours whiling away my time surfing the net. During that period of my life, my body felt more like a big burden rather than a blessing, and my enthusiasm for life itself understandably waned. Even though there was a part of me that *wanted* to take better care of my body and even appreciate it, I couldn't motivate myself to do so consistently. To make matters worse, I mistakenly believed that my dissatisfaction with my body would motivate me to stay more committed to my diets.

I bet you can't remember the last time you heard a woman say something wonderful about her body, such as: "I love my butt." "I look fantastic!" "Aren't my legs beautiful?" "Look at my full, luscious thighs." "My body is a work of art." Unfortunately, statements like these are as rare as finding a one hundred dollar bill lying unclaimed on a busy sidewalk.

Tragically and typically, you are *much* more likely to hear (or say) something along these lines: "Oh my God, I look horrible." "I'm so fat." "I've got to lose weight." "My butt is too big." "My breasts are too small." "I hate my stomach." "I'm disgusting." "I'm ashamed of myself." "I look huge in these pants."

We have become a nation of women who share a pervasive common bond of body dissatisfaction. And it's not just us grown *women*. The Dove Self-Esteem Fund did a recent study and discovered that ninety-one percent of *young girls* feel anxiety when they look in the mirror in the morning. Even adolescent girls are jumping on the body judgment bandwagon with forty-two percent of first–third grade girls wanting to be thinner. Unfortunately, our body dis-ease is contagious, and we are infecting our daughters. Surely we don't want to leave our children a psychological legacy in which they believe that being thin is more important than who they are and that their external appearance is more valuable than their internal riches. But that's exactly what's happening.

If we want to reverse the trend for ourselves—and for our children—we've got to *lead* by learning how to love our own bodies. Anyone who lives in this day and age knows it can be incredibly difficult to *like* your body, let alone love it. The "thinner is better" message is universally omnipresent in magazines, movies, television, on the Internet and in every other form of mass communication. There is such an obvious cultural bias towards one specific lean body type that we end up feeling inadequate because most of us do not look like the idealized super-skinny models in the ad campaigns or the celebrities we see in movies and on television. I'm of course not saying that thin bodies aren't beautiful, they are! But, I'm also saying that full ones are pretty too! *All* bodies have a beauty about them irrespective of their size. However, there are *very* few messages from the advertising and entertainment industry confirming this perspective. Instead commercial interests prey on our pocketbooks by selling to our insecurities. Although it may not be the advertisers' intention to make us feel bad about ourselves, the wave of negative body judgment they leave in the wake of their persuasive and misleading marketing pitches threatens to capsize our collective self-esteem. Their unrelenting emphasis on tiny bodies carries with it a potent and destructive byproduct for women in our culture.

Look, we all want to be thought of as attractive. It's human nature. So, if as individuals *and* as a culture, we are convinced that only one specific body type is desirable, we will, understandably, try to get as close as possible to matching that prototype, *even* if it means making ourselves miserable in the process. The insanely widespread nature of this cultural dis-order affirms and perpetuates the delusion that beauty comes in just one size and shape. And as a result, we buy into the "*only* thin is in" myth lock, stock and smoking barrel. There are very few voices of reason encouraging us to realize that beauty comes in an *infinite* number of forms and that inner beauty, expressed as a woman in a loving relationship with herself, is the most attractive quality of *all*. This is not some insincere drivel designed to trick you into feeling better about your current weight. It is simply the truth. Why is it, you ask, that a woman who is in love with herself and her body is the most attractive of all? Because her joy is utterly intoxicating. She glows with a powerful light from within that goes way beyond the physical. She projects a confidence and a zest for life that act as giant magnets, attracting both men and women alike. She sees her own unique beauty and everyone else does too!

A word about the men, ladies. I'm happy to share the fact that men are not *nearly* as picky about our bodies as we are, not even *close*. Yes, there is the occasional emotionally immature and shallow guy who is fixated on appearances. But in general, men are not *nearly* as obsessed with the size of our thighs as we are. We are holding *ourselves* emotionally hostage with the erroneous thought that we have to look like the women in movies and magazines to be thought attractive. When a woman loves her own body regardless of its size, and holds it in a respectful way, it is *massively* appealing to men. In fact a recent poll confirms, that the great majority of men do in fact love and appreciate full-figured women.

I wish I had known this early on in life. Before I healed my relationship with my body, I squandered massive amounts of energy doubting my attractiveness. My story is not at all unusual. A recent study indicates that nine out of ten women are dissatisfied with their bodies to some extent.

While there is absolutely nothing wrong with wanting to have a body that feels fit and healthy, one in which you feel attractive and vibrant, trust me when I say that disliking the one you have today will only push you further from your goal. For those who are choosing to release excess weight *because* they love themselves and because their health is being impacted, I support your intention wholeheartedly. I simply want to be sure you are armed with the healthiest approach available to assist you in meeting your goal.

Body rejection = Body disconnection = Compulsive eating =
Excess weight gain

Take a moment to contemplate your relationship with your own body. Has judging and disliking it *ever* helped you to release excess weight? I'm not just talking here about losing weight for a little while, but in the long term, has it helped you? Has beating yourself up over having gained weight made you feel better, more empowered, happier? Has comparing your body to someone else's helped you to create the body you want?

Are you closer to achieving your natural weight as a result of being hard on yourself? If you are like me, the answer to all of these questions is a resounding "No!"

When I started to respect my body and appreciate all the *good* things about it, even though I still considered myself "overweight" by societal standards, something inside me relaxed. I felt like I could breathe more deeply. I started to lighten up on myself, and voila, my eating habits became far less compulsive. I still had the desire to release weight, but I now knew that accepting my body would get me there faster.

Judgments of ourselves (although seemingly weaker because they are usually internalized) have a similar impact as when we are unkindly judged by someone else. Think of it in these terms: If someone you were close to told you outright, "Wow, you gained weight, and you look fat." "You look terrible." or "Yuck, those pants looks awful on you." you would probably feel shocked, awful and embarrassed. Although conversely, and unfortunately, you probably would not hesitate to look in the mirror and make those same harsh assessments of yourself. When you criticize yourself internally, you might not even notice it, even though on a subtle level it is making you feel deflated and depressed. When someone else criticizes you, however, you can't help but notice. It feels far more intense, like a slap in the face. You might protect yourself from the verbal abuse of others by walking away, or by insulting the other party in retaliation; however, it is rare for a person to protect herself from her own self-abusive thoughts, partially because our untamed mind does it so frequently that it's become status quo. And, because we do not fully comprehend how destructive and self-sabotaging it is, we continue to do it. Our inner critic is such a strong presence that we accept its barrage of insults without ever questioning it or attempting to shut down its tirades.

I'm here to tell you that no matter how insignificant a slight against yourself may seem in the moment, over time it not only tears away at your confidence but it will *also* notably depress your mood. If you shot an inflatable raft with a bullet from a gun, it would deflate rather quickly, right? If you continually poked tiny holes in it with a small safety pin, it would also deflate, just more gradually. The bullet is to the criticism from another what the pin is to criticism of yourself. One just deflates your self-esteem and mood at a slower rate, but either way, your boat is sinking. Each and every judgment you inflict on your body is like a puncture to your psyche that slowly but surely leaks and depletes your confidence and your enthusiasm for life and, understandably, increases your desire to eat for emotional comfort.

Learning to Accept Your Body

Let me be clear that learning to *accept* your body does not mean you can't also have an intention to achieve your ideal weight. Heavens no, that wouldn't have worked for me either! Rather, acceptance characterizes a *neutral* state of mind where you suspend judgment of your body in order to create a healthier relationship with it. You don't have to fall in love with it immediately, or think it is the most beautiful body you have ever seen, but be open to holding it in a place of respect and appreciation as you allow it to lead you to your natural weight. Your body is ultimately your best guide.

At one point in my recovery, the thought of accepting my body was frightening because I was worried I would lose my motivation to lose weight. My untamed mind convinced me that "acceptance" implied I didn't have the desire or drive to achieve my natural weight. This was obviously not the case. Acceptance and appreciation for your body is simply the *first* step towards enhancing your state of mind and consequently your ability to overcome the compulsion to eat when you are not hungry.

Again, this does not mean you have to pretend to be happy that you have gained excess weight or are carrying more weight than is healthy or natural for you. It simply means backing off of the really harsh and disempowering thoughts you hold about your body. This will open up a space for you to develop a stronger connection with your body that will allow you to achieve your natural weight. You don't have to like your body right away, but you *do* have to respect it and take care of it given that you will be spending the rest of your life in it.

To go directly from body rejection straight to body love was not possible for me. I had to ease myself into it over time as I learned how to shut down my untamed mind and suspend my body judgments as much as possible. If you are unable to access appreciation for your body right away, do as I did and make it your first goal to get to a "neutral" state of mind. All that a neutral body image requires is a *willingness* to respect your body now for the many wonderful ways it serves you. In a neutral state of mind, you perceive your body as neither good nor bad, but simply as a "fact," no different from the fact that your hair is brown, or your eyes are blue. Instead of thinking "I hate my arms," you redirect the thought to "Hey, that's my arm, I'm glad I have them so that I can pick up this bag of groceries." By neutralizing your negative self-judgments, you will diminish the shameful and frustrated feelings around your body that so often lead to emotional eating binges. Neutral is an early, but powerful healing stage.

Consider yourself involved in an intense, but gradual, courtship with your body. Remember, it takes time to establish trust in a new relationship, and developing faith in your body might not happen overnight. Keep in mind that the longer you have been neglecting and/or abusing your body, the more patient you have to be in your process of releasing old patterns and behaviors. There is a "getting to know you" period that must be expected and respected. Often the progression looks something like this:

Body judgment = High levels of compulsive eating

Neutral body image = Substantially reduced urges to binge

**Body Appreciation = Eating predominantly
in connection with your true hunger**

**Body Love = Eat solely to nourish and energize your body as you
please your palate**

Regardless of how dysfunctional your relationship with your body has been in the past, in this very moment, you have a chance for a fresh start. A "do over," if you will. Recognizing and owning all of your past body-rejection behaviors will be an integral part of your healing process and ultimately will be the springboard from which you can make far wiser choices. So let's gently review the past so we can create a better future.

Awareness Opportunity

The following exercise will support you in acknowledging where you are today in relationship with your body. Put a check mark next to any of the behaviors you currently do. Be compassionate with yourself as you review the list and remember that you are not alone.

Overeat and feel frustrated and depressed

Judge your body harshly

Feel ashamed of your body

Yo-yo diet

Compare your body to other bodies

Feel unattractive frequently

Eat when you are not hungry

Obsess over food

Experiment with diet drugs, laxatives and appetite suppressants

Feel "less than" because you can't lose weight on a diet

Starve yourself

Binge and purge

Obsess over the way you look

Eat to handle stress or any unwanted emotions

Compulsively overeat

Obsessively exercise

Believe only lean bodies are beautiful

Dread bathing suit season

Feel out of control around food

Sneak food because you are ashamed of your appetites

Distrust your body

Dislike your body

Eat to cope

Expect perfection of yourself

Think you should eat like other people

Feel ashamed to be seen eating

Deprive yourself of your favorite foods

Others ways you have rejected your body

Were you surprised by any of the behaviors you checked off?

Which of the behaviors do you feel most potently contribute to your unhappiness?

Can you imagine living a life free of these behaviors?

Don't allow your untamed mind to drive you to judge yourself for any of your past behaviors because up until now you were following the wrong map (diets and body judgment) as you were trying to get to the right place (body appreciation and living at your natural weight). We're trying to correct that now. We're switching tactics. Think of your budding partnership with your body as a brand new relationship. You might have the nervous jitters that accompany a new relationship you care about, or you might feel frightened because you are exploring new territory. That's normal. Just remember that building a healthy relationship takes place over time, and each new, positive experience will increase your confidence in your most trustworthy body.

So how *exactly* can you begin to form a healthier relationship or *friendship* with your body and make that transition from body judgment to body acceptance? Well, consider this.

Old thought cycle: *Negative body thought arises = creates disheartened mood = stimulates compulsive eating*

The diagram above illustrates the vicious cycle that results from negative thoughts about our bodies. As you can see, the very act of judging our bodies brings about or intensifies a compulsive relationship with food, and the outcome is excess weight, which, tragically, leads back to more body rejection. If you are one of the millions who has read Rhonda Byrne's best-selling book, *The Secret* or seen the independent film *"What the Bleep Do We Know?"* you are already aware that your *thoughts* create your *reality*. Both the book and movie explore the spiritual and scientific reasons as to why our thoughts are like powerful magnets, attracting that which we predominantly focus upon. So be smart about where you put your attention!

New thought cycle: *Negative body thought arises – Correct with a positive thought– Creates calm and centered emotional state – Binge urge dissipates*

When I started to correct my inner dialogue, my untamed mind would try to talk me out of honoring my body and myself. But I learned to ignore it and you will too! I have a friend who has named her untamed mind "Debbie," after a girl who was mean to her in high school. She gets particular pleasure out of saying, "That's enough, Debbie" whenever she is tempted to criticize herself. Sitting myself down and practicing slow and conscious breathing is what helps me to quiet down my untamed mind and shut out the judgments. I follow that up by speaking to myself kindly. You too will benefit from acknowledging yourself regardless of what your untamed mind is saying to stop you. Push past its voice of resistance. Think of your untamed mind as a pessimistic and negative friend you have to ignore because it ALWAYS gives you rotten advice, or the bully you must defeat in order to experience the life you most desire. *You can do it.* If you can think a thought, you can change a thought. You are in reality the author of all your thoughts.

Your Partner in Prime

Your body is your partner. The two of you are in a deeply committed, life long, primary, monogamous relationship. This relationship, like one with a best friend, spouse or significant other, has the potential to offer tremendous pleasure, joy and freedom, or if not properly cultivated and nurtured, it can create a great deal of frustration, anxiety and pain.

The best relationships are the ones in which the partners communicate openly and honestly, appreciate and acknowledge each other consistently and refrain from harsh criticisms. But how often do we *really* treat our bodies with such loving respect? When I was eating compulsively, I ignored my body's communications that screamed, "Enough, **Enough**, **ENOUGH**" when I was stuffing it silly. I failed to thank my body for all the miraculous things it does for me on a daily basis, and I disparaged it constantly. If I had treated a friend or romantic partner this way, I would have been one lonely lady. Not too many people would put up with that kind of conduct and still stay committed. But my body did, and your body does, each and every day of your life.

Luckily for you, your body is a forgiving, unconditional and perpetual source of love. This doesn't mean you're off the hook, though. If you had a husband or a boyfriend that you had a fight with and you *knew* you were in the wrong, that you had been really hard on him with no good reason, you'd probably want to make it up by apologizing and then being extra sweet and sensitive. If you have been intensely critical, neglectful or abusive towards your body, you now have a chance to "kiss and make up."

Maybe it would help if you heard your body's side of the story. If it could speak, your body might want to say something like this:

Dear _____ ,

I would like to formally introduce myself. I am your body. I have been with you since the moment you were conceived, and I have been with you through every single experience you have ever had. I am glad to have the opportunity to communicate with you directly because there are some things I have been wanting to tell you. The truth is that I am deeply frustrated with and saddened by our relationship.

You treat me poorly, both by neglecting me and judging me harshly, and yet you expect me to be energetic and healthy. I attempt to communicate with you all the time, but you don't listen to me. You ignore my signals that I have had enough food, yet you blame me for being overweight. You feed me when I'm not hungry and I have to work double time to process the extra food you eat. You know that exercise is good for me, and yet you make excuses as to why you can't fit it into your schedule. You know the foods that make me feel energetic, yet you choose to feed me in ways that actually inhibit my ability to be healthy, and then you are surprised and upset when you get sick. You tell me I am inadequate and that I don't look as attractive as you'd like me to be. Sometimes you compare me to others and then make me feel bad by telling me I don't measure up. You take the marvels of me, your body, for granted and instead focus on what you interpret as my imperfections.

As much as I love you, I must admit I am tired of being treated this way. It's gone on too long. If you treated anyone else the way you treat me, with a severe shortage of love and appreciation, they probably would not want to be a part of your life.

If you knew, really knew, all about me, you would feel great awe and appreciation for the miracle of nature that I am. My wisdom to support your survival and help you to thrive has been developed over hundreds of thousands of years.

If you listen to me, I can expertly guide you to excellent health. My instincts are infallible! No one knows what is better for your well-being than I do. I know the food, sleep and exercise routines that will provide you with optimal energy. I can also guide you to your ideal weight, and I can do it in a way that doesn't involve drugs, diets or extreme limitations. Once we are in communication again, we can explore all sorts of new ways to bring you pleasure.

I promise you that when our relationship is healthy, your life will be far less stressful and far more enjoyable. I realize that before now you didn't know that being unkind to me and judging me only made things harder on both of us, and I forgive you. Being frustrated with me clearly does not benefit you, or me, in any way, shape or form. We have the rest of our physical lives to explore and deepen our relationship. Let's make it the best that we possibly can, and remember, I want you to have it all. Make me your ally and there isn't anything we cannot have, do or be.

Love,

Your Body

<u>Awareness Opportunity</u>

Does this feel anything like what *your* body might want to say to you? Take a moment to write out what else your body might want to say to you.

Could you see loving your body with the same intensity that you do your pet? Or your child? Or the person that you love more than any other? That level of appreciation is available to you today. If you take a moment to contemplate what life would be like if you were you were faced with a chronic illness or even facing the possibility that you might lose a body part, a light-bulb might go off in your head illuminating the fact that having a healthy body is a true privilege. Try looking at it from this perspective for a reality check: If someone told you that you would have to have one or even both legs amputated because of a rare disease, do you think that any negative thoughts you had about your legs would be rapidly replaced with a huge desire to keep exactly what you had, regardless of their size or shape? You wouldn't care if you had cellulite; you would embrace your legs exactly as they are, most likely with a fanatical ardor. You might go directly from the untamed mind thought "I hate my legs" to the fervent prayer "Please, let me keep my wonderful legs." The thighs that seemed so unacceptable would become your object of deep appreciation. The threat of loss is a powerful perspective shifter that can turn down the volume on your untamed mind's continually dissatisfied diatribes about what you don't like about your body.

Together we are developing an understanding that it is the critical untamed mind, heavily swayed by cultural biases about what is the "right" body, that prevents us from appreciating our bodies now, in this moment. Appreciation for what you have allows you to have the centered state of mind that makes it easier to overcome binge eating. You would still be *you* even if you lost every part of your body except your vital organs, because you are far *more* than your body. That being said, your body is your carriage through life, your "ride" if you will, and the smartest thing you can do is take excellent care of it.

Your Natural Weight

Without exception, your body is your greatest ally and the most valuable physical asset that you will possess in the entirety of your life. Your only job is to appreciate it and take care of it as it directs you to your natural weight.

A word about your "natural weight." You have a genetic predisposition for a weight that will provide you with optimal health and vitality. You might have heard it referred to as your *set-point, ideal* or *natural weight*. Like your height or hair color, it is genetically predetermined. Your body will gravitate naturally toward it. Changing your natural weight is as impossible as changing your eye color or your ethnicity. It is your genetic design.

Just as no two personalities are alike, no two bodies are alike. If you try to fight your genetic design, you are signing up for major disappointment and frustration. Rejecting your natural weight or trying to achieve and maintain a weight that is beneath your natural weight will continue the spiral of body-rejection misery. Just as you would not try to fit your size eight foot into a size six shoe, trying to be a size eight when you are naturally a size ten is equally unrealistic. What this means is that your natural weight might not be what you previously set as your goal.

When I first read that my goal weight might not be my natural weight, and that I could not do anything to change it, I can remember feeling annoyed, defensive and, yeah, even a little angry. I did not want to be told that my goal weight was not possible and I was stubbornly resistant to opening myself to other options. Because I had not had a consistent experience of body acceptance in a long time, I could not even *begin* to picture embracing any weight other than the goal weight I was holding as "the ultimate." For a while I held on to that number like a hungry dog would a meaty bone, but eventually (I was a slow learner in this department) I saw that my attachment was preventing me from embracing my body as it was. So I let go and trusted that my body would lead me to the weight that was perfect for me, which, as is so often the case, within ten pounds of what I had envisioned. I knew my body was the ultimate authority on my health and I surrendered to its obvious wisdom.

Because I chose to care for and appreciate my body even *before* I reached my natural weight, I started to experience the joy of life more consistently. What I allowed myself to see, and genuinely believe, is that there is a beauty to EVERY body, each being appealing in its own unique way. I had several gorgeous full-figured friends who allowed me to see that feminine beauty comes in a multitude of forms, each having its own distinct appeal. My lovely *Rubenesque* friends held their bodies with supreme confidence and unquestionable assurance. And when I walked around with them, the appreciative glances and compliments they received made it obvious that others were highly attracted as well.

If your natural weight is fuller than the images put forth in the glamour magazines, you have a *great* deal of company. The average American woman is five feet, four inches tall and weighs one hundred forty pounds. The average American model is five feet, eleven inches and weighs one hundred and seventeen pounds. Most fashion models are thinner than ninety-eight percent of all American women. The lengths that some of the models go to maintain that super-thin body, verified by their personal admissions, are commonly unhealthy and oftentimes dangerous. Bingeing and purging, appetite suppressants, diuretics, compulsive exercise, self-starvation and smoking cigarettes are among some of the ways many of these ladies maintain their weight. It is a heavy price to pay. Attempting to stay at a weight that is not natural for you can cost you not only peace of mind, but possibly your health as well.

Hey, your goal weight might be your ideal weight. It's possible. Just be open to knowing that you can be as attractive and desirable at your natural weight as you would at the goal weight you have targeted. A tiny bit of willingness is all that is required. Your ideal weight might in fact be a few pounds lighter than you had envisioned or maybe a few pounds heavier. The key is to open your mind, just a teeny-tiny bit, to imagine the possibility that at your ideal weight, you will feel the self-esteem and feelings you currently associate with your goal weight.

If you *still* feel a little attachment to the goal weight you set for yourself, a powerful way to loosen and lessen it is by understanding that at your natural weight your body performs optimally. This means that at your ideal weight you will experience *optimum* health and the greatest degree of energy. You will also be less likely to get sick, and you may even extend your life. That's a bodacious bonus right there! Remember, your body knows best!

How will you know that you are at your natural weight? Your body will answer that question for you. Once you are eating in synchronicity with your *physical appetites* instead of eating out of habit or to escape your uncomfortable feelings, there will be a weight towards which your body will gravitate and then stabilize. At this weight you feel energetic and light and experience an "ahhhh yes, this feels right" intuition in your body. My experience has been that my weight stays within five pounds of my natural weight as long as I am *Eating in Alliance* with my true appetites. We'll learn more about natural weight and *Eating in Alliance* with your body in Chapter 5.

Your Body is a Genius

If you slow down and listen to your body, you'll find that it communicates to you through your feelings, both the delicious and the uncomfortable ones. When I feel good, physically and emotionally, it is a sign that I am making choices that serve me (e.g., endorphins after a workout, heightened energy after eating well, waking up feeling rested and refreshed, a rush of self-esteem after acknowledging myself). When I am feeling uncomfortable, the opposite is usually true.

Your body often attempts to attract your attention through discomfort, prompting you to "wake up" to a behavior, a thought or a choice that is not serving you. It will give you a stomachache if you overstuff it or possibly a headache if you are working too hard and running yourself ragged. It will only tolerate so much unhealthy behavior on your part before it steps in and "complains" by creating some form of anxiety, tension, pain or illness, encouraging and inciting you to make some shifts. If it could speak to you directly about what it most wants *from* you, here's what your body would most likely want to say:

Message From Your Body

Dear_____,

Here are some of the ways you can show me that you love and honor me, not necessarily in this order, but all of them are important to me. I love to get enough rest, to get to bed early enough so that I can wake up slowly and I work best when sleeping in synchronicity with Mother Nature's rhythms, which means earlier to bed, earlier to rise. I realize that this can't always be honored, but it is my preference. Not getting enough sleep makes me cranky, makes it harder for me to concentrate and wears down my immune system and therefore my ability to fend off illness. Even if you think you are a "night owl," please do your best to try to get me to bed earlier.

Nothing sets a better tone for the day than when I make the transition from the dream world to real life in a gentle, nurturing manner. I really appreciate it when you invite me to start the day with either meditation, journaling, inspirational reading and/or a few minutes of luxurious stretching rather than anxiously rushing me out of bed after the alarm clock rings and putting me straight to work. That's a pretty harsh way to start the day.

Next, I humbly request that you feed me as many healthy, whole, live (straight from the earth) foods as possible. Something that is either plucked from a tree or harvested from the ground. These are a "10" for me in terms of maintaining high energy and health.

Please listen to me when I tell you I have had enough to eat—

overstuffing simply wears me out. And if you have gained excess weight, please don't be mad at me and judge me unkindly. That works against our efforts to release any weight you put on when you ignored my signals for "full." I appreciate the fact that you want me to maintain a weight that is optimal for my health and well-being, but if you are abusing me in order to make this happen (i.e., dieting, appetite suppressants, chronically fasting, purging), you are defeating the purpose of your intention. Please try to accept me as I am today even if your intention is to achieve your ideal weight. Resisting my current weight and shape will only make things worse. Resistance only exacerbates your frustration and fires up emotional hungers. If you accept the weight I carry today gracefully and temporarily, it will help dramatically. If you love me and listen to me, together we can release any extra weight gained through emotional eating.

Be sure to take me out for some form of exercise at least four times a week for 30 minutes or more and please include both some form of stretching (yoga is one of my favorites) and some form of cardio vascular activity. When my heart rate goes up, I breathe more deeply, which acts as an instant stress reliever for both of us. Exercise is not only one of the most powerful things you can do to ensure my consistent health, but it is also a de-stressing, anti-aging, immune-boosting practice. On top of all of those benefits, it is a natural high. Remember how alive we feel when those endorphins are released? I want more natural highs!

Also, just like "man's best friend," I love being outside. Take me outdoors at least once or twice a day and go for a leisurely stroll or just hang out on a park bench or some other place you find beautiful. I thrive on fresh air (and getting in and out of the car running errands doesn't count). In many cases, depression is related to spending far too much time indoors, it is just not natural or healthy. The more time we spend in Mother Nature, the happier we'll be. This I can guarantee.

Something else that helps me to thrive is drinking water. I want at least four glasses a day, and more if possible. Other liquids don't count because water does a better job, more so than any other beverage, of oxygenating my cells. When my cells are oxygenated, I have far more energy. Water also flushes out toxins and slows my aging process. It will be easier for you to stop eating compulsively if I am properly hydrated because you won't confuse my being thirsty with my being hungry.

And by the way, I know it's really fun, and I don't want to bring the party down, but alcohol is a depressant. Use it consciously with this fact in mind. The same recommendation applies to caffeine and processed sugar, both of which give me a temporary boost but deplete me in the long run. Choose a healthier alternative whenever possible (e.g., water, a walk, fresh fruit). Obviously you don't have to cut any of them out entirely if you don't want to, but do your best to make them treats as opposed to staples of your diet.

Regardless of my weight, hold me with pride by practicing good posture. It will make you feel better to stand up straight with your shoulders back and your spine erect not only because it indicates a respect for yourself and me, but also because when you are standing this way, I can work in the most optimum fashion. When you go from a slouching or hunching-forward position to an upright one, my lung capacity is increased and this allows me to breathe more deeply, creating a relaxed feeling for us as well as a natural high.

Last but not least, if I am sending you signals that I am uncomfortable or tense, do not avoid the feelings but rather explore them. Listen intently to determine what it is I am trying to share with you. Perhaps I am guiding you to lighten up on yourself, or to move on from a situation that is not serving you. Maybe I am encouraging you to take a break in the middle of the day. Once you slow down and connect with my wisdom you will find I am a brilliant life coach. Deep breathing can support you and me in working through and diffusing your difficult feelings with greater ease. It also relaxes me more than virtually any other activity, so practice tapping into your breath throughout the day to minimize anxiety, access the joy of the present moment and quiet the illusory thoughts of the untamed mind.

Thank you for taking the time to hear my side of the story. Clearly I have your best interests at heart because my purpose is to support you in having the healthiest and most joy-filled life possible. Partnering with me will be one of the smartest things you have ever done. Remember, I'm your buddy!

Sincerely and Lovingly and All Ways,

Your Body

Now that your body has an opportunity to talk to you about what it wants, it's time to create a new relationship with it by thinking differently *about* it and acting differently *towards* it. The new body appreciation paradigm will look something like this.

Old Pattern	New Pattern
Dieting	Eating in alliance with your body
Hating your body	Accepting/loving your body
Weighing yourself	Throwing away the scale
Eating for emotional reasons	Eating when you are hungry
Exercising compulsively	Exercising for health and fun
Eating compulsively or impulsively	Eating slowly and consciously
Comparing your body to others	Loving the body you are in
Judging and disliking your body	Loving your body
Getting dehydrated	Drinking 4–8 glasses of water
Repeating history	Creating a new reality

It doesn't take a rocket scientist or a Rhodes Scholar to see that the new reality you are creating for yourself is not only far healthier, but also far smarter. Each of the behaviors affiliated with the new paradigm adds to the quality of your connection with your body. Even *little* changes in your behaviors will make a large difference over time. Tiny shifts build on each other, like compound interest in your bank account. Keep in mind that even if you improve your thinking, about yourself and your body, one percent each day, *you will be one hundred percent better in one hundred days*. For this reason, congratulate yourself with uninhibited enthusiasm for even a one percent improvement.

Now take a moment to wrap your arms around yourself and send the most loving thought you can think of to your body. Promise your body that "things are gonna change" now that you understand what a sacred temple you possess and that you will honor it on entirely new levels. This, my friend, is the beginning of a beautiful love affair.

Now close your eyes for a moment and envision a world where women love and accept their bodies in the fantastic variety of shapes and sizes they assume. This new world is being born, one woman at a time, starting with *you*. You will be one of the "pioneers," creating a new model for future generations by loving your body. It's a powerful purpose to focus on, and you'll be making the world a sweeter place by committing to it. Once you start to inhabit your body with genuine love and appreciation, you will come to find that it is the vehicle through which you can and will experience new levels of delicious pleasure, mind-blowing fun and outright bliss. It is a joy ride just waiting for you to take the wheel!

*****

"Problems cannot be solved at the same level of awareness that created them."

- Albert Einstein

Chapter 4

The Power of Your Beliefs:
How Your Thoughts Impact Your Emotional Appetites

We've explored many of the physical and mental reasons why diets don't work no matter how faithfully you follow them. We've talked about how loving your magnificent body and yourself are both vital to the process of releasing excess weight. Now it's time to delve even deeper into some of the very specific *beliefs* that may be keeping you stuck in a compulsive relationship with food.

The truth is if you're like I was, and like so many other women are, you probably do eat more food than your body needs. Time after time, even though you desperately want to shed those extra pounds, something drives you to eat that extra helping of pasta or just one more piece of cake. You want to be fit and healthy, but sometimes it just feels impossible to stop eating. Is it just a lack of willpower?

Of course it's not. In the moment when you make the decision to eat or not to eat, it is not just about the food. You do not eat compulsively solely because food tastes good, and certainly not only because your body needs more fuel to keep going. There are a variety of very powerful *emotional* factors that drive the compulsion to overeat that are directly stimulated by the *beliefs* you hold. These beliefs are usually related to fears and worries of your untamed mind and they drive your emotional hungers.

Once you identify what I refer to as your "binge-inducing beliefs," and create healthier beliefs that are empowering to you, you will be able to create a healthier relationship with food and with your body. Here's where you get to spend some time reflecting on your past, going within to determine the origins of your lack of appreciation for yourself and the incidents that made you feel bad about yourself. Perhaps "going within" and reflecting on your fears and self-doubt doesn't sound very appealing to you. Maybe you would prefer to let sleeping dogs lie and to avoid looking at the more painful moments in your past. I can understand that. It can be hard emotional work. But here's the deal. If you don't figure out what *specifically* is causing you to overeat when you're not hungry, it is very likely that you will stay stuck in the same vicious cycle. You can't move beyond your compulsive eating if you don't know what is at the root of it.

Once you discover what specific emotional issues and beliefs are sabotaging your relationship with your body *and* learn to deal effectively with the challenging emotions that you are attempting to avoid by eating, your "emotional" appetites will dwindle dramatically, freeing you from an endless focus on food. That, my friend, is most certainly worth the trade-off. The answers to all your questions about how to overcome compulsive eating and what is driving your emotional appetites lie in a very sacred space—in you.

The University of You

Whether you know it not, there is far, far more to you than you currently realize. Chances are excellent that you are more focused on a narrow vision of who you are, the micro version rather than the macro. You, like the majority of us, have your eye trained more towards what you are not than all that you are.

This is why it so very crucial to do inner discovery work. It is the door through which you can contemplate yourself with far greater depth, far greater accuracy and far more compassion and appreciation. If you don't explore your inner realms, your deepest dimensions, you will see only a limited perspective of your true essence, the very surface synopsis of you. Consequently, you won't be fully aware of the inner resources you possess that will allow you to conquer your compulsion with food and get more of what you want out of life, whether it's a healthy relationship, a career you are passionate about, great friends or financial abundance that allows you to have more freedom or fun in your life. Self-awareness is the foundation upon which you can build your dream life. It helps you to develop the understanding that you are the "dream operator."

In the following pages you'll find the support you need to begin your own exploration of the influences and beliefs that drive your emotional appetites. In some cases, you are going to be returning to your earliest memories. This may bring up some tender emotions. Admittedly, my own path to greater levels of self-awareness was not always an easy one. I had to face some emotions and experiences that I had avoided *precisely* because they were difficult to face. I had little desire to dredge up my past to find out what was at the core of my eating issues, but the alternative was to stay stuck where I was, which was no longer an option for me because I was making myself so incredibly miserable. There were moments of great sadness as I came to grips with how deeply down the path of self-abuse I had traveled. I also experienced moments of intense anger in which I blamed my parents and society for my sorry plight as well as moments of anxiety and huge frustration as I struggled to incorporate new ways of interacting with food and viewing my life and myself. But there were also many more moments of tremendous relief and joy when I was *finally* able to see clearly what was preventing me from finding peace around food.

I would have done the personal work *much* sooner had I realized that the process wasn't nearly as bad as I thought it was going to be and that my emotions, although intense, wouldn't swallow me alive or overwhelm me totally.

Does freedom from worry and excess stress, from doubting yourself, from unnecessary fears about the future sound good to you? Great! Then start getting ready for your journey within. The path to self-awareness requires "grace and grit" to trudge to the top, and you may have to fight the urge to turn on your heels and head back down the mountain when the going gets tough. But, when you reach a peak moment of awareness and self-acceptance during your climb, you'll see spectacular views of a life that was unimaginable when you were standing at the bottom of the hill. That's what makes it all worthwhile, and you have everything it takes to get there! You have the courage; you have the strength; you have the curiosity (I know this because you bought this book), and you have the right intention–to accept your body as you achieve your natural weight.

In the following questionnaire, you will be exploring your personal history to gain insight into the individuals and the experiences that have contributed to your current sense of yourself and your relationship with food. Through the questionnaire, you'll be reviewing your past to see how it is influencing your present. One of the goals of this exercise is to become even more intimate with yourself than you are today, to go deeper with yourself than you ever have before! So be totally honest when answering these questions, no one will see your answers but you. It represents a wonderful opportunity for you to see the "movie" of your life more clearly so you can then start to create more of the happy scenes you deserve.

Awareness Opportunity

I invite you to find a quiet and peaceful place and answer the following questions. Leave yourself enough time (thirty minutes or more) to spend with the questions so you can dig into the most vivid memories you possess. Make sure you are alone in a cozy and comfortable place that feels safe to you. Play some soft music you love in the background. The more relaxed you are, the easier it is to access your subconscious mind and your earliest memories. As you write your answers, allow yourself to do so without questioning your thoughts. Write down the first ones that pop into your mind. Remember that there are not right or wrong answers here, only memories, beliefs and feelings that are true for you. The only perspective to consider and honor in this particular exercise is your own.

Part One: General

At what age did you start to become aware of different body shapes and sizes?

1-8   9-16   17-25   26-35   36-45   46-55   56-65   Over 65

At what age did you remember starting to judge your body?

1-8   9-16   17-25   26-35   36-45   46-55   56-65   Over 66

When you were a child (4–12) did you consider yourself:

Underweight   Optimum Weight   Overweight

Do you remember being at peace with your body at any time in your life? If yes, circle the ages that apply.

0-5   6-11   12-16   17-22   23-30   31-40   41-50   51 or above

At what age did you go on your first diet?

Who were the other people in your life who influenced your relationship with your body? (e.g., teachers, siblings, friends)

What events in your childhood made a deep impression on you?

Part Two: Family

If you were a foster child or had stepparents, please answer the following questions with them in mind.

What was your impression of your father's weight when you were a child?

What was your impression of your father's relationship with his body?

Did your father ever make comments about your body?

What was your impression of your mother's weight when you were a child?

What was your impression of your mother's relationship with her body?

Do you remember being treated with great respect by your parents?

When you acted out as a child, how did your parents discipline you?

Did you feel safe sharing your fears or worries with your parents?

Did you feel you were highly valued by your parents?

Do you remember feeling embarrassed by the way your parents reacted to you at any time?

Did you feel your father was preoccupied or present when you were a child?

Did you feel your mother was preoccupied or present when you were a child?

What happy events stand out for you in your early childhood?

What traumatic, shaming or unhappy events stand out for you?

Part Three: Sexual Activity

I have included quite a few questions about early sexual experiences because eating disorders are common among children who were sexually abused or raped. It is an incredibly tragic and common experience. One out of every six American women will be the victim of a rape or an attempted rape during her lifetime. Fifteen percent of these victims will be under the age of 12. If you were sexually abused as a child, the most loving thing you can do for yourself is to get some support in the form of counseling. Be gentle with yourself as you explore this highly sensitive topic. If you feel overwhelmed as you are answering the questions, listen to your heart and stop. Return to this section when you feel you are in the appropriate space to handle the emotions that accompany looking back on painful memories.

Do you remember having any sensual or sexual activity in your childhood?

At what age did you become sexually/sensually active by choice?

Were you ever inappropriately touched, sexually abused or raped by anyone in your immediate or extended family?

Were you ever inappropriately touched, sexually abused or raped by a stranger, a family acquaintance or a date?

Was your first sexual/sensual experience a pleasurable one?

Do you have any regrets about your first sexual/sensual experience?

Was there a relative in your life or any individual in your life who was sexually inappropriate with you at any time in your life?

What were the messages you got in your household about sex?

Do you feel any of your sexual experiences influence your relationship with food today?

Part Four: Summary

If you read your entire self-inventory as though it were someone else's, what would you say were the major contributing factors to that person's current relationship with her body?

Which of your answers surprised you?

Oftentimes compulsive overeaters are able to identify specific events or experiences in their formative years that caused them to disconnect from their bodies. Some women are able to relate their rejection of their body with some harmful sexual experience. Others can relate it to being shamed by one or both parents in regards to their blossoming sexuality. Some individuals can relate it to the need to be perfect for their parents or suffer the consequences of their wrath. These are just a few of an enormous number of variables that contribute to the complexity of a compulsive relationship with food. As children, our innocent hearts and developing minds sometimes interpreted events in magnified ways because we were so pure and vulnerable. It is important that you allow yourself the freedom of seeing how big each childhood event was for you, even if as an adult you feel you might have blown it out of proportion. Becoming intimate with the "story of you" will allow you to develop new levels of compassion with yourself that will in turn lead to a diminishing emotional appetite.

After completing this exercise, you might see some patterns that originated in your childhood that are still influencing your relationship with yourself and your body today. You might also have a stronger understanding of how deeply influenced you were by your parents and early role models, recognizing that you adapted and adopted some of their attitudes and beliefs, some of which are not serving you. The ones that are holding you back from being happy are the ones we are going to address next.

This written exercise might have revealed to you particular incidents you had suppressed because they were so highly painful. Shining the light on them by revisiting them might stir up some strong emotions. I encourage you with all of my being to seek support and guidance in the form of therapy if your childhood held high levels of abuse or neglect. This road is best traveled with a loving support structure to ease you through the process. Going it alone can be incredibly difficult and confusing and it can also delay your healing process dramatically. If I could go back and do it all over again, I would have submerged myself in my healing and gotten as much help as possible early on so that I didn't have to suffer so long. Don't create optional stress for yourself by putting it off. Be smart and be brave and get the support you deserve! Knowing about the incidents and experiences that contributed to your current relationship with yourself and your body is different than healing them. In my case it took both time and therapy to move beyond my old hurts. I gave myself the gift of patience during my process and it proved very healing. I encourage you to do the same. Therapy will help you learn how to give to your inner child today what you most wanted in your childhood, whether that was loving attention or stronger boundaries. Nurturing your inner child will be a tremendous act of self-love and remember, each self-loving behavior takes you one step closer to not only your ideal weight but also to the life you dream of!

The Influence of Childhood Messages

Many of us feel as though our lives fall short of what we would like them to be. We have a yearning in our hearts to feel fulfilled and joyous, safe and carefree. We want to be happy, but we are not sure how to make that happen consistently. After years of immersing myself in the study of happiness, not only *how* to be happy, but what keeps us mere mortals from experiencing happiness consistently, I found, not surprisingly, that *the most important factor* was, as we reviewed in Chapter 3, the relationship that each of us has with ourselves. The answer to the unhappiness that accompanies self-doubt is...drum roll please...self-love. It is the "Holy Grail," the Mount Everest and the gold medal of personal achievements. And yet true self-love is a precious but incredibly rare condition in this world.

You may not even be quite sure *why* you don't value yourself highly, or why you feel convinced at times that you are "less than" others. What you *do* know is that there are times when you feel unworthy and unlovable.

Why is this? Why would you, or any one of us, doubt our own value? What stands in the way of our feeling appreciation and respect for ourselves? Why do we judge ourselves so brutally, compare ourselves to others and believe we don't measure up?

The fact of the matter is that we were *all* born with the capacity to feel good about ourselves, to genuinely like, honor and respect ourselves. That ability, however, can be diminished by negative messages—some intentional, others unintentional—that we received from a parent (primary caretaker) or authority figure (teachers, relatives, etc.) early in life. Our childhood experiences and the way we were treated as children *greatly* influence our self-esteem (or lack thereof). While nature (genetic makeup) most certainly plays a substantial role in determining our personalities and character, parental influences play an equally powerful part. If you were treated predominantly with love, respect and gentleness as a child, you are more likely to treat yourself in the same way as an adult. If the opposite was true and you were treated disrespectfully, unkindly and unfairly, you would be more prone to treating yourself in a similar fashion. Because of their innocent and open nature, children are highly influenced by early programming. They are open books with their parents' writing on their unfilled pages. Children, of course, frequently believe that their parents have all the answers to life and are accurate in their beliefs. Generally your parents have the greatest influence over your beliefs, not just the beliefs you have about life in general (religion, politics, prejudices, values) but the beliefs you hold about yourself as well.

In the above awareness exercise, you might have remembered some painful incidents from childhood and/or recalled some of the ways you were treated as a child that left wounds on your tender heart. Most of us were not parented perfectly, probably because most parents receive no training before entering into the toughest (albeit most rewarding) endeavor of all time. Most people have no *idea* what they are signing up for when they welcome a new life into the world. Crankiness, exhaustion, anger, intense frustration and overwhelm show up frequently, and because many parents lack the skills to calm themselves by shutting down their untamed minds, the children take the brunt of their emotions.

If, somewhere in your childhood, your parents or someone you loved very deeply made you believe something was "wrong" with you, that you were a "bad" girl, or even if they didn't seem very interested in you or seemed annoyed by you, it negatively impacted your self-esteem, and may continue to trouble you today. Whether it was delivered through a spanking, unkind words, an unfair punishment or even a menacing glance, acts of emotional hostility, impatience, disinterest and anger towards a child are intensely influential to their tender psyches. You might even have accidentally or unintentionally been sent the message that you were inadequate, selfish, stupid, not good enough, lazy, unattractive, a burden, uninteresting or inferior by your parent(s). But unintentional or not, messages from the authority figures in your life impacted how you see yourself today.

Even if you received many *positive* messages from your parents, even if your parents loved you more than anything in the world and gave you a secure and happy childhood in many wonderful ways as mine did, the experiences that made you feel ashamed, inadequate, embarrassed, isolated, unloved or unworthy still had an emotional impact. Was it safe for you to express your anger as a child? If there was no place to express your anger, it is likely that you would turn it on yourself. Were you able to express your sadness to your parents and feel like you were honored for your feelings and shown compassion and sympathy? If it was not safe to express your sadness, food might be the way that you choose to avoid your grief today. If you were made to feel your feelings were not as important as those of your parents, it is not surprising that you too would learn to ignore them.

The negative messages we received in childhood often become internalized as part of the image we carry of ourselves and color our sense of self-worth so that we believe we truly are unworthy, unattractive or simply not good enough. These negative beliefs can trigger feelings of shame, sadness or inadequacy that are always lying just beneath the surface, ready to bubble up when we're stressed, tired, hurt, angry or frightened and in some cases, even when things are going unusually well.

Compulsive overeating is one of the many faces of addiction. Children who were neglected or treated unkindly or disrespectfully often turn to addiction as adults to quell the feelings of inadequacy that constantly threaten to rise up and overwhelm them. Those of us who feel we "lack" something often eat as a way to replace the "bad" feelings of insecurity and worry with the distracting pleasure of eating. We may turn to food in an attempt to keep those feelings and negative self-judgments submerged and to numb ourselves from the great discomfort of facing them. But like a big beach ball that you try to push under water, there is a force that constantly drives the fearful and self-defeating thoughts to the surface.

But wait. If these disempowering thoughts are there all the time, why aren't you aware of them? The problem may be that you've been listening to the negative voice in your head for so long that you barely notice it anymore, and when you do, it is so upsetting and depressing that you attempt to drown it out by turning to food. These insidious negative thoughts can be so quietly and subtly delivered that they simply escape your notice, like the faintest of whispers. But you will know when that negative internal dialogue is taking place because you will *feel* some form of discomfort. You might not always catch your self-defeating thoughts, *but you will always catch your feelings if you are paying attention.* A nerve-wracking inner dialogue creates the desire to escape, and food becomes your drug of choice. Who can blame you? Nobody wants to constantly hear negative and harsh feedback; it is disheartening and offensive. So shutting down that voice inside your head through eating becomes your main coping mechanism. The louder and more

129

negative your inner dialogue is, the greater the urges you will have to eat compulsively.

As we learned in the meditation exercise in Chapter 3, your thoughts are flowing nonstop, like a perpetually running loop of tape, chattering away at the prompting of your untamed mind all day every day, erroneously suggesting that you are somehow inadequate (e.g., "You look fat in those pants." "She looks so much better than you do." "Get a hold of yourself and stop eating." "What is wrong with you?") or getting you to doubt your abilities (e.g., "You didn't do that very well." or "You didn't get enough done."). The untamed mind also whiles away the hours by getting you to worry about something that might or might not happen (e.g., "You're going to be late." "You have too much to do, you'll never finish."). While some of the time the inner critic is so quiet and subtle it doesn't grab your attention, at other times it is as loud as an oncoming locomotive's whistle, you just can't miss it. Your inner critic is your most ruthless judge, and it has the power to make you feel miserable. The steady stream of negativity it feeds you is as harmful as hooking yourself up to an I.V. of liquid depression, which is why it is so important to practice observing the inner dialogue running on those tapes, so that you can stop the low-vibration suggestions of your untamed mind that are sabotaging your happiness. Observing and raising the bar on your inner dialogue, as we covered in Chapter 3, is a key part of your self-love practice. As you do it, the feelings of inadequacy, shame or anxiety will dissipate, and you'll be able to let go of the need to bury them with food. You will be learning how to access the kinder and gentler voice in your head, the one that will consistently make you feel empowered rather than tense, so you won't have the constant compulsion to eat. The following section will support you in becoming more intimate with how your mind works so you can harness its potential and make it work for you rather against you!

The Influence of Subconscious Beliefs

You are probably already aware that you have a conscious and subconscious mind. But just for clarity's sake, I'll make a simple distinction between the two. Your *conscious* mind holds the beliefs and experiences that are really familiar to you, the content of your life that is "fresh" in your mind. Like really close friends, the beliefs and memories of your conscious mind are well-known to you. If your conscious mind holds the vividly known and easily recalled memories, your subconscious holds the vague or long-forgotten ones. In other words, if your conscious mind represents your *best friends*, your subconscious mind represents your *distant relatives*.

Your *subconscious* mind is the giant warehouse that holds *all* of your beliefs and life experiences in tremendous detail. Like belongings that have been packed away in an attic so long that you forgot you had them, many of your experiences and beliefs have been in "storage" in your subconscious.

Although you are not familiar with all the beliefs and past experiences in your subconscious mind, they can, and do, influence your behavior. If you eat compulsively and you don't know why, your subconscious mind holds many of the answers for you.

Many of my own subconscious beliefs were based on the thoughts that I was not good enough, but I had *absolutely no idea* that these beliefs resided in my subconscious mind! If you would have asked me, I would have said that much of the time I felt pretty good about myself. But my compulsion around food indicated otherwise. Although I thought *consciously* that I was a good person much of the time, my treatment of myself on a day-to-day basis was predominantly harsh and sabotaging. Strangely, even though I always felt self-conscious, I never would have believed I had very low self-esteem. I wouldn't have believed that I disliked myself, even though I rarely acknowledged any of my accomplishments and was constantly judging myself. I was woefully unaware of how hard I was on myself because it had become so habitual. The negative voice in my head was so loud at some points that I frantically tried to drown it out through food so that I couldn't hear it. I believe that is part of the reason I wasn't completely tuned in to how unhappy I was. I was too numbed by the food binges. Compulsive eating allowed me to push the "mute" button on my emotions, both the bad and the good. It was usually only in moments of deep crisis or depression that I was able to see clearly how dire things had gotten, how unhealthy my behaviors were.

Driven by my emotional pain, I started asking myself deeper questions (e.g., Why am I so hard on myself?) in order to figure out where my reoccurring sense of inadequacy was coming from. Asking myself intimate and searching questions allowed me to dip into the recesses of my subconscious mind where I found some disempowering beliefs about myself. This is part of the reason that therapy is so helpful, because you get an opportunity to dig around in your subconscious mind and contemplate yourself and your life on a more intimate level. You get to find out what items in the "storage" unit called the subconscious need to be discarded. What really helped me turn the corner and accept the fact that I had some negative subconscious beliefs "running the show" of my life is when I stopped eating long enough to pay attention to my thoughts, to "witness" them like an outside observer. Instead of eating compulsively when I was stressed, I started to sit myself down and breathe deeply to relax myself as I pinpointed the untamed mind thoughts that got my emotional hungers raging. As I started tuning into my thoughts with far greater consistency, it allowed me to see how frequently I was thinking of myself in an unkind, impatient and unforgiving way. Prior to that point, although my untamed mind could be very hard on me, I was not aware of the buried subconscious beliefs fueling the negativity. I wasn't really at the wheel of the car I was driving through life, I just thought I was! Through therapy and self-reflection, I was able to see how some of my childhood experiences, long forgotten consciously, negatively impacted my self-esteem, and were driving some of my emotional hungers.

When you were filling out the prior questionnaire, you might have come across an old sad or unhappy memory you hadn't thought about in a long time. It was there of course, but there was no reason to dredge it up and think about it before now. But it was there in your subconscious mind nonetheless, hanging out like an unwanted guest.

Your conscious mind holds ten percent of your beliefs and memories, whereas your subconscious holds up to ninety percent. If those submerged beliefs are impacting your life, it is clear that it would help to know what they are. If you had a house that had termites that, if left unchecked, could take the entire house down, you'd want to do the work to get rid of them. The same is true of the disempowering thoughts in the subconscious mind. You want to do the emotional work to find out what and where they are so that you can rid yourself of them. Knowing what's going on inside your mind will allow you to do a little housekeeping to ensure that you keep the quality, high-vibration beliefs and throw the rest out with the garbage.

Here's a very specific example of how the subconscious mind can influence your life. Let's say I consciously believe that being thin will make me happier, and in spite of that desire I constantly make choices that sabotage my intention to release excess weight. Chances are good that there is a competing belief in my *subconscious* mind that is even more powerful than the one in my *conscious* mind. That belief might be that if I am thin, something else might go wrong that would be even worse. It might be that I'll be threatening to people I love if I am thin. (We'll be reviewing specific disempowering beliefs that often lie at the heart of eating compulsions later in this chapter.) Once you identify the negative or disempowering beliefs in your subconscious mind, you will be able to choose to change them, but again, you can't change them if you are not even aware that they are there!

You would think that because you are *thinking* your own thoughts, you would already be savvy to *how* you are thinking, but strangely enough that's not always the case. We're usually too busy thinking our thoughts to notice them or to give them specific attention. We'll often listen more closely to other people's thoughts than our own. We humans are a funny lot! When you really start to zero in on your specific thoughts and beliefs, you may be surprised (as almost everyone is) to see how many of them are not serving you.

Freeing Yourself from Your Fearful Thoughts

When fears are abundant in your conscious and subconscious mind, they create anxiety and unhappiness and prevent you from being in the moment and relaxing and enjoying life. Let's be honest, who can be truly happy when they are tense or frightened? You may be thinking, "But I'm not a fearful person by nature," and that may very well be true. However, I'm not talking here about the "scary movie" kind of fear where you are terrified or horror-struck. I'm talking about the subtle and general fears that far more frequently show up as worry, insecurity and anxiety.

How often are you afraid that you are never going to lose weight? How often are you worried that something bad might happen? Or that something good that you really *want* to happen might not? How often do you experience anxiety about what others think about you? Most of us spend so much time worrying about the future that our present moments are riddled with anxiety, which is why we'll reach for a donut when what we really need is to be reassured around our fears. The more fear you have, the more likely you are to struggle with addiction because most addictions are attempts to escape from our fears. Are you worried much of the time? Then it is a sure sign that there are subconscious fears and, more specifically fear-driven *beliefs* to be discovered and eliminated.

What is a Belief?

Although I have always had a general understanding of what a *belief* is, I'd never really taken the time to consider my own, to reflect on them individually to assess their value and veracity. I had my beliefs, I thought they were valid, and that was pretty much that…or so I thought. I didn't realize how influential my beliefs are and I certainly was not aware of the fact that my fear-driven beliefs were at the root of my compulsion around food. We'll get to that in a minute, but first I want to familiarize you with how your beliefs are creating your reality.

We can define a belief as a *strongly held perspective, an acceptance by our mind that a thought is true or real, which is often accompanied by an emotional sense of certainty*. That sense of certainty makes us accept our beliefs, or perhaps cling to them, even when they are not completely true! An example of one of the disempowering beliefs I held was "I'm not attractive unless I'm thin." Although it was not true, I *believed* it without reservation and, unfortunately, I had that emotional sense of certainty that accompanies a belief. The truth was, I *was* attractive in my fuller body, but my belief was so strong that I couldn't see myself clearly. This is just one example of how a belief can wreak havoc on your self-esteem.

A belief starts out as a single simple *thought*, but when we think that same single thought over and over again, it becomes a *belief*. If I think the thought "I'm an unattractive person" just once, I might not *really* believe it entirely. But if I say it to myself repeatedly, it enters the "belief" department of my untamed mind and becomes a highly influential force. You can see why being aware of your thoughts is so important because if you are repeating the low-vibration ones, you are more deeply imbedding a disempowering belief in your psyche.

Let's take it a step further. Your thoughts, repeated, become your beliefs, and your beliefs determine how you feel and your feelings prompt your behaviors.

Thoughts (Beliefs) - Will Incite Feelings - Will Incite Behaviors

I can remember looking in the mirror– and thinking– "No one is going to love me when my body is this big." Over time my belief became "Because I'm overweight, no one will find me attractive," and as a result my feelings were depression and hopelessness. I attempted to escape the discomfort of those feelings by eating compulsively (behavior). My negative thoughts and beliefs triggered intense negative feelings. The feelings, because they felt so overpowering, brought me down, like a rock tied to my leg in a lake. When I repeatedly ran that negative thought through my mind, *that's* when I reached for food to try to make the bad feelings go away.

Now mind you, this little mental saga was often running just beneath the surface of my awareness. I wasn't paying attention to what I was thinking back then, so much of the time I didn't understand what made me hypnotically head for the kitchen. What I did know was that I went into autopilot, eating whenever I felt bad. It never occurred to me to trace my uncomfortable feelings back to the low-vibration or fearful thought that was upsetting me so much that I would try to drown it out with food.

There are many fear-driven beliefs that are common among compulsive overeaters. In this chapter, your assignment, should you choose to accept it, is to figure out which ones you have been holding onto so you can let go of the ones that are driving your urges to eat when you are not hungry.

It is your turn and great opportunity to now choose your beliefs based upon what feels right and true to you today and to correct the old, sabotaging beliefs that have been holding you back. As you read the forthcoming list of detrimental beliefs, you might pinpoint some instantly as those passed down to you from your parents or another adult authority figure. Others may seem only vaguely familiar, but still push a big emotional button for you. Pay attention to your *feelings*! They will help you to determine the beliefs you have bought into and the ones that are low-vibration. Those that are limiting, self-sacrificing, fear-driven or judgmental will feel bad. Your uncomfortable feelings are your body and soul's way of saying, "Let go of this one, my friend."

Remember, once you identify the disempowering beliefs you hold, you can change them. You hold the controls. You are in charge. You are the captain of your destiny, charting a new life for yourself. Fortunately, you will be able to shift some of your beliefs quickly. You'll quickly see their debilitating and limiting nature and something will "click" in your tamed mind that will allow you to let it go faster than a hot coal. Others, because they have been a part of your psyche for so long, will shift more gradually. If you have held a belief for a long time, it sometimes takes some effort to change it. But the more you focus on a healthier and more empowered belief to replace the old one, the faster your behaviors will shift to align with the upgraded belief.

Think of adopting a new belief and its related behavior as planting a seed and watching it grow into a tiny sprig, form a bud and finally, burst into a lovely flower. That's how the new belief birthing process works. All you need to do is:

1. Be willing to let go of any belief or behavior that doesn't serve you.

2. Think of a thought/belief that feels more loving and supportive to you than its predecessor.

3. Repeat the new thought/belief to yourself as frequently as possible, especially when the old belief runs across your untamed mind.

You obviously can't force a bud to bloom faster than is natural, but you can create the optimum conditions for the flowering to take place by focusing your attention on the healthiest and highest vibration thoughts you can imagine. The more consistently you recognize and correct the unhealthy beliefs you have that are related to yourself and your body, the more you will eat because you are physically hungry rather than emotionally distraught. The more you focus on the higher vibration belief you come up with to disarm the old disempowering one, the easier it is to soften the feelings of stress, insecurity and fear you have been trying to avoid.

Awareness Exercise

Throughout the following section put a check mark next to any of the low- vibration beliefs that you can identify with on any level. There are alternative healthy beliefs listed after each bogus belief, a higher vibration perspective, for your consideration. I invite you to give each higher vibration belief a test run by speaking them out loud to see how they feel in your body. If you can come up with one that feels more empowering to you, *that's* the one to focus on!

I'm Wasteful if I Don't Eat Everything on My Plate

The "Clean Plate Complex" is a common theme in many homes. When I was growing up, I couldn't leave the table until I had finished my entire meal (or at least the majority of it). I was a particularly skinny child with a pretty small appetite, and my mother, in her genuine desire to make sure I was healthy, made it a personal quest that I eat almost every morsel on my plate before I left the dinner table. She regrets it now because she understands the ramifications of pushing me to eat when I was not hungry. At the time, however, she was afraid I would get sick if I didn't eat the food she had made for me, so she was very strict about making sure I ate my entire meal.

My mother also knew that I had an intense sweet tooth, so there was a pretty good chance I had snacked on something sweet at my friend Helen's house after school. This made her even more determined to make me eat the healthy food she had prepared. Oftentimes I would sit at the table for what seemed like an eternity, pushing my remaining scraps around my plate, long after my three sisters had finished their meals and were off playing games, doing homework or watching television. I would frequently sit at the table bored, ignored and lonely, feeling stuffed and trying to force myself to shove in the last bites of my dinner.

I figured out pretty fast that finishing everything on my plate would make my mother happy, so I started ignoring my body's signals for "full" or "satisfied," a learned pattern that became progressively worse later in life. This led to many years of overeating as I continued to disregard my body's communications long after I was no longer living with my mom. Finishing my entire plate even when really full became a habit that slid right into my adult life and stayed firmly engrained until I discovered a new belief that served my relationship with food and my body. This new belief was "I only eat what I am hungry for and I stop when I am satisfied."

In other homes, the "Clean Plate Complex" stems from a parental desire to make sure their children understand that not all people have access to regular meals and that inadequate distribution of food and starvation are very real problems. The "children are starving all over the world" argument often contributes to guilt-driven eating. I'm of course not advocating wasting food. However, given that eating disorders can result from forcing children to eat when they are not hungry, this is not the best way to solve the world hunger problem. It goes without saying that when your child eats their entire meal, it does nothing to actually put food on a hungry child's plate. Food drives and volunteering at a food bank are powerful ways to encourage a child to understand the predicament of the poorest of families without compromising their relationship with their body.

Awareness Opportunity

Were you told to finish everything on your plate as a child?

Do you have a compulsion to clean your plate at every meal?

Did you ever eat more than you were hungry for because you felt guilty or wanted to please a parent?

If you have the following "old belief," see if you can replace it by repeating and internalizing the "new belief" suggested below.

Old Belief: *If I don't finish everything on my plate, I am selfish/wasteful.*

New Belief: *I listen to my body and I eat until I am satisfied. If there is food left over, I feel free to turn it down or save it for another time or day knowing that this is the best choice I can make for my body.*

Eating Three Meals a Day is Vital to My Health

Do you eat three times a day even if you are not hungry? Do you find yourself getting up in the morning and pouring yourself that bowl of cereal, or scrambling up those eggs, even when you are not getting any hunger signals from your body? Most of us do. Why? Well partially because that's what everyone else does too. It is simply the cultural norm. Breakfast, lunch and dinner were unquestioningly a constant in my home growing up and as a general rule we all ate together and we rarely skipped a meal. Which was fine in theory, except there were many times that I ate not because I was hungry, but rather because it was a designated mealtime.

Eating out of custom rather than out of legitimate hunger is quite common. We eat not because our stomach is grumbling and our craving for food is strong, but instead because breakfast is being served, or dinner is already on the table. While set mealtimes are a tradition that can be bonding and healthy experiences, when you have a compulsive relationship with food, eating for any reason other than because you are physically hungry is not advisable if you want to stay connected with your body. Just because it is your normal breakfast time doesn't necessarily mean it is time to eat!

For years, even when I was not hungry for breakfast, or lunch, or dinner, I ate out of my ingrained belief and assumption that it was the "right" way to eat. Engaging in the ritual of dining at certain times of the day was a habit I found to be challenging to break simply because I had been eating that way almost my entire life. I often felt deprived when I didn't eat a meal, even when I wasn't hungry. Heaven forbid I should miss dinner! It wasn't until I finally realized that eating in synchronicity with my true hunger felt so much better on so many levels than eating out of habit that I was able to make the shift away from eating simply because it was dinner, or lunch, or whatever!

Looking back, I can see that it was even easier for me to justify my compulsive eating when it was mealtime. "I should eat," my untamed mind would say, "it's breakfast and they *say* that breakfast is the most important meal of the day." Or, "It's dinner time so I'll eat this healthy meal of spinach, whole grain pasta and grated organic cheese, even though I'm not hungry, because it's good for me." Observing my attachment to mealtimes and becoming aware of my tendency to ignore my body and give in to my desire to eat with other people was a light-bulb moment for me. I realized I had fallen prey to the cultural norm to eat at designated times. I'm most certainly not saying don't eat breakfast, lunch and dinner, I do almost every single day. But when I was first starting to learn new ways to listen to my body, I had to be flexible. There were times when I had eaten a big lunch and wasn't hungry at dinnertime, but was really hungry around 9:00 pm. If I had eaten earlier, I would have been eating *out* of concert with my body. Waiting until my hunger kicked in allowed me to re-sync with my appetites, and that, my friend, is when I started releasing excess weight.

By all means, if you are hungry four, five, six or even seven times a day, eat and enjoy! Remember, your body is *totally* unique. It is an original. It may be that for you to have optimal health and energy, five small meals a day may be more appropriate for you than three meals. With experimentation and time, you will come to find what is right and true for you and your body. No one knows what is better for you than your body does. Listen up and lighten up!

Awareness Opportunity

Were you told that it was healthy for you to eat three meals a day?

Was it a pattern or ritual in your home?

Can you see value in eating when you are hungry as opposed to on a predetermined schedule?

Old Belief: *I should eat breakfast, lunch and dinner every day for my health.*

New Belief: *Mealtime is anytime my body is hungry.*

I Should Eat Now Because I Might Get Hungry Later

Preventative, or pre-emptive eating takes place any time you eat *before* you are hungry because you think you might not "make it" to the next meal without getting *extremely* hungry. I know from experience that the "extremely hungry" feeling can bring up a lot of angst, almost a suffocating sensation of overwhelm. Many people eat breakfast because they are afraid they won't "make it" to lunch. They snack now, even though they are not getting any hunger signals, because they are going to be at their son's baseball game all day and don't know when they will

145

eat next. Or they'll be in meetings at work and might not be able to eat for hours.

These are understandable motivations and concerns because, yes, there is a chance that you might not feel hungry now, but might be ravenous in an hour. However, this form of pre-emptive eating is like filling your gas tank when it is already on full. In order to stop yourself from having to eat in *anticipation* of not being able to eat later, you have alternative options available to you. One technique I use is to bring a snack with me as I'm leaving my house and eat it when I feel my true hunger signals coming up. I almost always have some dry roasted almonds in my car in case I get a hunger urge and I'm unable to stop and eat. If I want to be hungry at dinnertime because I know there is a delicious meal ahead, I'll eat just a little bit, enough to curb my hunger until then. It means a little extra effort on my part to pack a snack or even take my meal "to go," but eating in synchronization with my body brings me such pleasure that it is well worth it! I now take a doggy bag with glee!

Having made mental notes, and scribbled notes in my journal about my typical eating habits, I understand my body and food patterns well enough to know that if I eat a big dinner, I am rarely hungry first thing in the morning. In the same way, if I eat a light dinner, I am usually very hungry early in the morning. If you would like to gain a stronger perspective on your own eating patterns, write down what you eat. It is a potent self-awareness exercise that will serve you powerfully.

Awareness Opportunity

Do you ever eat because you are worried about not having access to food later?

Are you comfortable feeling hungry?

What's the worst thing that can happen if you get that hungry feeling?

Old Belief: *It is better for me to eat before I get hungry because I might not have access to food later, or the time to eat later, when I am busy.*

New Belief: *I wait to eat until my body is hungry knowing that it is optimal for my weight, health and energy levels.*

I Should Eat to Please Someone Other Than Myself

Are you eating to please someone other than yourself? Did you as a child? "Pleaser Eating" sometimes originates in a household where hard-working, dedicated moms and dads cook meals that take significant thought, time and energy to prepare. After slaving over a hot stove, let's face it, they might enjoy being appreciated for their efforts, and as a child, you may have obliged them by eating when you weren't hungry.

But the "pleasing" eating mode isn't confined to your parents' home. It also takes place when you eat at someone else's home, perhaps a friend's house, and you eat far beyond what is comfortable to acknowledge the chef for his/her efforts. Socially it is seen as a compliment when you eat everything on your plate, but if it is at the expense of staying connected with your body, it is *never* okay. I don't care if your host is your boss or

147

the President of the United States; there is no justification for overeating to please someone else. You can always ask your host to serve you smaller portions so that you can honor your body and the chef at the same time.

Recognizing that there still might be a part of you that is looking to "please" by eating can be a major step in putting a stop to a compulsive relationship with food. I eat because it is pleasurable and because I want to nourish and energize my body. I know it is okay to turn down an offer of food from *anyone* under *any* circumstances. Heck, I wouldn't want anyone to eat just to make *me* happy no matter how much time I put into preparing a meal, and I assume the same is true of any of my friends.

Awareness Opportunity

Was there someone who was made to feel good because you enjoyed their cooking?

Who might you be eating for today?

Would you want someone to eat to please you if it meant they were being untrue to, or sabotaging himself or herself in some way?

Old Belief: *If I eat everything on my plate, I can avoid hurting other people's feelings or feel like I am "good."*

New Belief: *I eat to please myself and nourish my body.*

I'll Feel Less Stressed If I Eat Something

In times of stress, food is frequently the "drug of choice" to diminish anxiety. Stress eating occurs when a specific event, an ongoing situation or an individual is "hanging out in your head," prompting your untamed mind to cause you undue anxiety or frustration, which you attempt to divert through a delicious snack. I used to eat to avoid digging in to large work projects, paying bills or even cleaning my house. The more stressed I felt about the work in front of me, the more I wanted to eat. I didn't know how to access the reasonable, patient, tamed part of my mind that would tell me, "Hey, just relax; take a deep breath. If you take one small step at a time, it will all get done. It always does…remember?" Instead, I let my untamed mind run amuck and always went looking for a distraction in my pantry.

You may be using food as an avoidance mechanism, to calm the feelings of discomfort that are running through your body or to manage stressful events or relationships in your life. But you now know that eating to avoid stress is like trying to put out a fire with lighter fluid. That is why it is important to become an expert in untamed mind muzzling. This skill will give you the calm feeling you are looking for without the remorse that dependably follows compulsive eating. Chapter 8 details specific empowering, relaxing and centering tools that will provide you with nurturing alternatives to compulsive eating in times of stress.

Defining your specific high-likelihood stressors can be helpful because you'll be able to identify and prepare for the times when you are more likely to want to overeat. Is it at the end of the day when you are bored

149

with the thought of doing the dishes? Is it before going to your in-laws' house or your parents' house? Is it when you are alone at night?

One of the things I do when I observe my untamed mind doing its dance of delusion is to have a gentle conversation with myself. I deal well with stressful situations by talking tenderly to myself while exploring options to any challenge I am facing. I was a *big*-time stress eater, and even today I am extra mindful during hectic times to be sure I'm not using food to diminish the tension I'm feeling. I used to believe that dealing directly with a stressful situation would be far more difficult than eating a Twix candy bar and ignoring my plight. But this ignorance did not lead to bliss because it turned out the exact *opposite* was true! Facing discomfort and exploring options leads directly to some level of resolution, providing me with a feeling of peace I was looking for in the food I was eating. I now ask myself powerful questions designed to get to the heart of what's bothering me rather than skirting the issue through food. For example, I might ask myself, "Hey, what's bothering you?" "Why are you so tense?" "What can I do to calm and reassure you that it is all going to be okay?" When I answer these questions, I can feel my capacity to breathe expanding, my stress dropping and my understanding growing. From this place I can relax, think clearly and choose an alternative to food to deal with my stress.

Awareness Opportunity

What situation feels overwhelming to you in this moment?

When are the times you are most likely to want to eat compulsively?

What alternatives do you have to deal with stress in a way that will ultimately bring you peace of mind?

Old Belief: *Eating helps me to reduce my stress and cope with my problems.*

New Belief: *When I eat in harmony with my true appetites, my stress levels decrease dramatically and I can deal with my emotions in a responsive way.*

I'm Afraid to Succeed

Abraham Maslow, author of *Toward a Psychology of Being*, had it right when he said, "We are generally afraid to be that which we glimpse in our most perfect moments." Many of us are afraid of our tremendous potential, our divinity, our light, our unlimited capacity to create success in our lives. Whereas it does, of course, seem highly appealing to be successful on some levels (the financial rewards, the positive attention, the freedom), many of us anticipate that it carries with it the additional weight of responsibility, accountability, stress and excess attention. For some of us, it is much easier to hang out in a state of life uniformity, where the highs aren't too high and the lows are bearable, than it is to "go for the gold."

Success opens up a whole can of worms of new experiences and opportunities, which inevitably means change of some sort, and the untamed mind struggles mightily with change. Change, even if it accompanies achievement, is still a form of the unknown to the untamed mind, which adds a certain level of psychological turmoil. As we all know, turmoil is never the smooth ride we pleasure-seeking animals prefer. Any time we stretch outside of our emotional comfort zones, the untamed mind gets busy coming up with umpteen reasons to worry. For example: Even though we may be unhappy with our current weight, we all know there is a certain level of comfort in staying in a situation that feels familiar. For some of us, being thin represents the "unknown," which generates all sorts of fears. The untamed mind prefers the predictable, the knowable, the sure thing. The unknown is an incredibly scary place for most human beings, even when staying where we are is tremendously unappealing.

You may have a subconscious fear of losing weight because you are concerned it will bring up a whole new host of situations that will be stressful. You may wonder, "Will I receive unwanted interest from men? Will people expect more out of me? Will I have to reject and hurt someone who is attracted to me? Will others be envious of me?" Again, the untamed mind can run amuck with imaginary fears about the pitfalls of success. This is what keeps us stuck in unhealthy eating behaviors that paralyze our progress. Many of us, quite frankly, would rather "deal with the devil we know" (excess weight), rather than the "devil we don't" (our lives at our natural weight).

I never thought that I would be afraid of something as pleasurable as success. In fact on many levels, I yearned for it. But, in retrospect, underlying my desire to be successful, I had some beliefs about what I perceived as a high-achievement life that made me uncomfortable. One of these beliefs was that if I became highly successful, I would have farther to fall. In that way, the fear of success also includes a fear of failure.

The higher I climbed the ladder of success, the more risk I imagined I was taking. Who knew what could happen if everything was going fantastically in my life? My untamed mind had a field day coming up with "worst case scenarios" about what could go "wrong" if I was successful. The thought of it made me feel vulnerable. Vulnerable not only to unforeseen challenges that I anticipated might accompany the attainment of my most ardent dreams, but also to what others would think and feel. Did I deserve success? Was I smart enough? Hard-working enough? Even when it came to my body, I thought that living at my natural weight, which I saw as a successful achievement, made me even more exposed. My extra weight felt like a cushion, a barrier (albeit a phantom one) to my imaginary fears, but it also held me back from my true potential because I couldn't navigate life with ease physically or emotionally. I had to be willing to feel my fears and take action to move towards my goals in spite of my untamed mind. I want to share a powerful perspective with you: It is a lot easier to embrace success when you know how to calm your untamed mind and access the truth–your success, your happiness makes the world a better place.

One woman I had a coaching relationship with expressed a fear that, if she didn't have her weight problem, some other much larger problem would come up, like someone in her family would get cancer or she might get in an accident of some sort and get seriously injured. (My God,

153

that untamed mind is fertile!) This fear-driven belief kept her hooked in a highly compulsive relationship with food. Like this woman, your fears may not be rational; nonetheless, they *feel* very real to you. So it follows that if you don't address them and leave them unexplored and unhealed, they will act as a barrier to your growth and weight-release efforts. You've got to investigate each one, each limiting fearful thought you have about succeeding, like a math problem. Spend time figuring out where the fears came from, be with the fear and revisit it so that its silly nature becomes obvious to you. Greet the disempowering thought/belief head-on. When it shows up, say, "Hello. There you are again. What are you trying to tell me? Don't worry so much, there's nothing to be afraid of."

If you experienced uncertainty and a lack of consistency in your childhood, where parents were attentive and gentle one moment and unkind or insensitive the next, it can sometimes be difficult to trust that life can or should be consistently joyous. You may find that when your life is going smoothly and you are experiencing great success in some area that you have an accompanying fear that it will all be taken away, or some misfortune will befall you. The fear that the "other shoe is going to drop" is understandable because of the emotional instability that a small child experiences if a parent is loving with them one moment and then turns on them aggressively in a moment of anger. If this was the case for you, you may feel like you walk on eggshells in your life, worried about your future, living with repetitious question of "What if (insert misfortune here) happens?"

This is why creating the safe internal space that we discussed in Chapter 3 is so important. It is the ideal place to take yourself when you are worried that things might go wrong. It is the place to go when you want to be reassured. When life throws you a curve ball and something challenging is happening, you will have that space to turn to calm you so that you can find a high-vibration perspective on what you are facing. Treating yourself with loving compassion can help to reduce the fear that something bad might happen.

Awareness Opportunity

What are you afraid might happen if you achieve your natural weight?

How do you define success?

Why might you be afraid of success?

Old Belief: *If things are too good, something else might go wrong. No one gets to have it all, and I might not be able to handle the stress that comes with success.*

New Belief: *Joy, peace and abundance are my birthright. I know that the entire Universe is conspiring with me to have my heart's desire and all I have to do is love myself and enjoy the success I was meant to have.*

If I Eat I'll Feel Less Lonely

When I did not know how to love myself, I often felt very lonely. Although I had a large circle of phenomenal friends, three amazing sisters, two wonderful parents and eleven nieces and nephews I adored, I still felt an inner emptiness that couldn't be filled no matter how big my community. I didn't feel empty all the time; I had a very active social life and busy career. But the times when I was at home by myself, *especially* after attending a big party with lots of couples, the vacant feeling would return. Because I didn't like feeling lonely, I ate to drive the feeling away. I'd head straight for the kitchen where I knew my friend, food, lived. Then I'd grab the remote control and turn on my other "friend," television, and hang out with both of them until, full to the brim, I would force myself to go to bed.

For some of us, feeling lonely is so overwhelming that we, understandably, attempt to "stuff" the feeling down with food to reduce its intensity. And yes, food does mute the uncomfortable feelings a bit, but we all know it only does so in the short term. If you are not getting the love you desire, food often becomes an improvised or makeshift companion. This is reasonable, as we are social beings and the desire to feel a connection is entirely natural. However, when the connection with food damages your connection with yourself and your body, the cycle has to be broken. Helping you to learn how to fill yourself emotionally, by appreciating yourself fully, is one of the intentions of this book.

How can you fill that empty space within? I have two techniques. One is to find ways to spend time with myself that are nurturing and fun. The other is to tenderly talk to myself when I feel lonely, to connect with my inner child who always longs to be reassured, to coach myself kindly. An important belief that assisted me in engaging in these two behaviors came when I finally understood and embraced the fact that the Divine always loves me unconditionally and eternally. This lovely and comforting belief dramatically diminished my "lonely eating" patterns. Once you absorb this truth, whether you are a religious person or not, the same will be true for you!

Awareness Opportunity

When do you feel the loneliest?

What do you do to diminish your loneliness?

How would you nurture a friend who felt lonely?

Old Belief: *If I eat, I won't feel as lonely.*

New Belief: *I eat to nourish my body and if I am feeling lonely I talk gently to that part of myself that has forgotten that I am loved unconditionally by the source that has created everything I know and love.*

I Might Get Hurt If I Get Too Close to Someone Else

While some compulsive eaters use food as a way to take care of themselves when they are feeling lonely, others use it to protect themselves from getting too close to someone. They maintain excess weight as a barrier to intimacy. Loneliness may be difficult, but rejection for some is much tougher because it feels so personal, like someone has stripped you down to your birthday suit, taken a good hard look and then walked away. It can knock the wind out of your mental sails.

For years I can remember appeasing my wounded ego when a man I liked wasn't romantically attracted to me by citing my weight as the culprit. "He'd like me if I were thin," I'd reassure myself, thereby softening the blow of rejection. I actually appreciated having the weight excuse as my default excuse. I could handle the rejection of my body, which I also judged as too big, but I couldn't handle what I perceived as a rejection of *myself*. I didn't understand at the time that just because someone was not interested in me it didn't mean I wasn't desirable. It just meant that person was not a match for me, we simply were not meant to be together. I also didn't realize that if there wasn't a connection for the guy I was interested in, it merely meant there was someone better out there for me. Rather, I took a lack of interest very personally. My extra weight was an emotional buffer that I relied upon.

Many women put on excess weight as a way to isolate themselves from the pain of rejection and, in the process, have inadvertently created a lonely existence for themselves. If in childhood you perceived that your love was rejected, it would not be surprising if you attempted to protect yourself in the only way you knew at the time, by holding onto excess weight. The problem with this strategy is that by trying to *avoid* pain, you inadvertently end up *creating* it for yourself. The barrier to feeling hurt by some phantom partner or friend in the future becomes the pain we live with today. We hurt ourselves in the moment in anticipation of the hurt that might come in the future. Now is the time in which to be daring. To take a chance on the joys that are available to you by "cowgirling" up and riding the thoughts of your untamed mind into submission so that you can get over wanting and wishing for intimacy– and start having it! And remember…it's a self-loving act to put more importance on what "you" think of you over what "they" think of you!

Awareness Opportunity

Do you feel excess weight keeps you safe from rejection?

Do you feel more comfortable with life when you are fuller figured?

Is intimacy something you embrace or something you avoid?

Old Belief: *Being overweight prevents me from getting hurt.*

New Belief: *I am safe at any weight because I can always rely on myself to be loving, compassionate, gentle and present.*

I Don't Want to be a Threat to Those I Love

When I first achieved my natural weight, I had a few friends who had a difficult time adjusting to the leaner me. When one of my friends told me she had a hard time being around the skinnier me, I was deeply hurt at first, surprised and sad. And then I got angry, *really* angry. I knew that she knew how much I wanted to be thin and how I was always struggling in my relationship with food, and she could clearly see how much happier and healthier I was living at my natural weight. I was disappointed that she couldn't find it in her heart to be glad for me. I had never been competitive or envious of her, even though she was adorable in every way so I couldn't understand why she could not feel happy for me. I took it as a sign that she didn't really care about me. I found myself eating compulsively to manage the strong emotions I had around her reaction to my body and, of course, I started gaining some weight back. In retrospect I can see that I sabotaged myself because I was afraid of losing my friend, a friend I cherished deeply, who felt like a sister to me.

With time and understanding, I ultimately came to realize that her inability to be happy for me didn't mean she didn't care for me deeply. She was simply listening to her untamed mind, which spurred on a competitive and insecure inner dialogue. She had not yet developed a loving relationship with herself, one in which she could see her own incomparable beauty so that she would feel no need to compare herself with me. I understand that now, and I wish I did then, too, because I think it could have healed the friendship.

One of the reasons it is so important for you to love yourself is because women who have learned to love themselves are able to genuinely revel in the success and happiness of other women. They can offer friendship in its highest form. And healthy friendship is one of the *most* joyous and healing energies on the planet. It is a source of guidance, compassion, love and nurturing. It's one of life's greatest gifts. The purpose of friendship is to share the joy of life, to support one another in seeing your respective magnificence, to help each other create lives you are passionate about and, of course, to have as much fun as possible while you are growing and learning along with life.

While I always hold a space for friends to come back into my life after a falling out, my choice is to spend my time with people who are in healthy relationship with themselves so I don't have to hold myself back in any way for fear that I will lose their friendship. Fear-driven eating patterns can stem from the belief that if you are too magnificent, too thin, too funny, too smart, too beautiful or "too anything," others will be threatened by you. Yes, it is true that there are some women who have a difficult time embracing a woman in love with herself. But not so with all women, and those are the ones you want to hang with! The ones who want the very best for you!

For me, if jealousy and envy exist in any friendship, they undermine the relationship. This is true even if my friend is a close relative. Do you have a friend who makes you feel unsupported and uncomfortable? It is important to carefully consider those you spend time with because they impact you in many ways. It is worth taking time to clearly define the purpose of your friendships. If your friend attempts to sabotage your happiness because she feels inadequate, you have the option of setting a boundary to limit your interactions or even to put the relationship on hold until she is able to see her own unique beauty and consequently able to fully embrace yours.

I'm sensitive to the big-hearted and forgiving woman out there who doesn't want to lose a family connection or a friendship, especially one that she has had for a long time. However, it is a profound act of self-love to surround yourself in your innermost circle with people who are committed to supporting you in having the best life experience possible. Having to downplay your own magnificence or feel guilty because you are enjoying life will sabotage your efforts to live life to the fullest. Remember, this life isn't a test lap, it's the grand prix!

Holding yourself back is not only damaging to you, but it is not supporting your friend. Truthfully, holding yourself back, or trying to appear less happy than you are, only enables your friend to stay in their "stuck" position with you paralyzed right along with them. Base your friendships on unconditional love, mutual respect, enormous support, uninhibited fun, committed service and true celebration. Don't be afraid to create a temporary separation with those friends who attempt to sabotage your happiness or make you feel guilty for having joy. I guarantee, when you truly love yourself, you will attract people who are capable of offering true friendship and they will be as devoted to your joy as you are. You deserve only the best.

Awareness Opportunity

What is your purpose for friendship?

Which friends/family members are unable to share your joy today?

If you sensed someone in your inner circle was envious, would you feel comfortable confronting them or creating temporary separation?

Old Belief: *If I am too successful, then (insert name here) will not want to be around me.*

New Belief: *I allow myself to be all I can be, knowing that my true loved ones will celebrate my every happiness.*

162

I Want to Lose Weight So I'll Be Attractive to Others

Many women attempt to release weight so that they will be acceptable to "other" people in their lives (parent, boyfriend, relative). Do you have someone in your life who is constantly riding you to release excess weight? Someone who attempts to control what you eat? Perhaps you are afraid that if you are not thin, you will lose the love, attention or respect of someone that you care about. Maybe you are afraid that someone will be angry or upset with you for not matching his or her ideal.

Attempting to release weight with this specific fear as an incentive is a *huge* block to successful weight release, and it virtually guarantees compulsive eating, I know it, I did it! Any time your incentive to be thin is related to someone else's desire, you will be drawn towards overeating. The pressure will drive you to it; the disempowered purpose will stimulate the urge to binge.

Your efforts to release weight cannot be for *anyone* but yourself. Why? Because somewhere deep inside, in the innermost part of your being, you know that it is unhealthy if someone is withholding love from you if you are not fitting their "image" or "picture" of what you could or should look like. That's not how real love works.

The purpose of intimate relationships is to share the joy of life, to experience unconditional love and mutual support. This doesn't mean you have to break up with the boyfriend who is encouraging you to lose weight, or cut off communication with the mother who tries to tell you what to eat, it just means you would benefit from creating some healthy boundaries around what is acceptable behavior if you choose to stay in relationship with them. Being goaded, teased, manipulated or punished by a significant other because of what you weigh is abuse–even if that person tells you they have your best interests at heart on some level.

Is there anyone you know who wants you to lose weight as much as you do? It's unlikely. So clearly someone else putting their two cents in about your body without your permission merely makes you feel more pressured and instigates more compulsive eating. I had several boyfriends who were invested in my losing weight; it had nothing to do with me being healthy and everything to do with my looking the way they wanted. Because I couldn't accept my own body, it was not surprising that I would draw in someone who had issues with my body; they were merely reflecting my own lack of self-acceptance.

When I finally committed to achieving my natural weight, it was for me, not for anyone else. Thanks to the powers that be, I also learned to value myself enough to choose men who appreciate me for who I *am* rather than just what I *look* like. Just like me, your beauty transcends your physicality, and becoming aware of this fact will allow you to exude that loveliness to all who are graced to be a part of your life. Know that you are lovable and desirable exactly as you are today, without changing a thing.

Awareness Opportunity

Is there anyone in your life who is going overboard in their efforts to get you to lose weight?

Is that relationship supporting your intention to love yourself?

What action step can you take or boundary (loving guideline) can you make with anyone in your life who is pressuring you to lose weight?

Old Belief: *I have to lose weight for others to love me and find me attractive.*

New Belief: *I choose to take care of my body and release excess weight so I can have an experience of health and lightness. I choose to spend time with those who see my beauty at any weight and love me just as I am.*

I Can Escape My Frustration By Eating

Following college, I started out in a career that I knew wasn't right for me. I took a job selling copy machines not because I had any interest in them, but because my close friend Amy had a job there and we thought it would be a blast to work together. Well, it turned out that it wasn't nearly as much fun as we thought it was going to be. Selling copiers door-to-door in office buildings was a really hard sell, and often an exercise in futility, and most certainly an exercise in humility given the number of doors I had slammed in my face. I dreaded going to work, but I couldn't get the motivation to research other job opportunities, and I didn't slow down long enough to contemplate what career would make me happy.

After attending a self-awareness workshop, I learned a valuable perspective and made an important distinction for myself. I realized that a "job" is something you do to earn money. Whereas a "career" is a way to support yourself while doing something you love. My frustration eating diminished dramatically when I went to work for the Leukemia Society and was engaged in work where I felt like I was making a positive difference in the world.

The truth is that your soul, which is intimately connected to the Divine, wants you to have an experience of joy every single day, and until you take action to change the areas of your life that are causing you constant angst, you will continue to receive the "gift" of your frustrated, dissatisfied and grumpy feelings to prod you to take some action.

It works the same way in frustrating relationships. If you feel unheard, unappreciated or misunderstood by your partner, food often becomes a consolation prize. When you find yourself in a relationship in which you experience the same frustrations over and over, it is a sure sign that there is something wanting to be discovered and healed. Frustration with another often indicates an area where you are being guided to learn how to give to yourself what you are seeking from someone else.

For example, in my past I attracted men who rarely complimented me, even when I bent over backwards to please them. I felt frustrated with their lack of attentiveness, but I didn't know how to ask for it without appearing needy. My aggravation with them drove me within myself to discover why I kept attracting men who took advantage of my giving nature. What I came to discover is that I needed to learn how to genuinely value myself, to compliment myself on things I did well or even appreciate myself for my efforts before I could anticipate that gift from anyone else. Again, my frustration eating diminished as I stopped playing a victim and figured out what *I* needed to feel good rather than waiting for anyone else to give it to me!

Awareness Opportunity

What quality (attention, affection, appreciation, acknowledgement, understanding) are you looking for in your partner/ parent/employer/sibling/friend that you haven't yet learned to give to yourself?

What frustration has been showing up in your life consistently?

What action step(s) can you take to move beyond it?

Old Belief*: Eating will help me feel less frustrated.*

New Belief: *I face my frustrations head-on by considering my options and taking action in the areas where aggravation repeatedly shows up to urge me to make some changes.*

Food Is the Greatest Pleasure Available to Me Today

Many spectacular women are living lives that lack the passion they crave. Because they do not yet have an understanding of their own infinite ability to create anything they want in their life, and because their lives are not matching their expectations for joy, they seek pleasure through food. Are you lingering in a job you are dissatisfied with, a relationship that is unfulfilling? Are you forgetting to make time to pursue activities or hobbies that you feel excited about? If your answers are yes, then consider it a waving red flag that you are wanting some pleasure! It is no wonder you would reach for the "sure thing" in the form of a Twinkie or a bowl of pasta.

But the problem is that the "sure thing" makes life much worse when we use it as a substitute for the "real thing." And, to quote Marvin Gaye, "There ain't nothing like the real thing, baby!" By making choices to stay with any situation, personally or professionally, that doesn't feel right in your heart, you have unintentionally limited your pleasure potential. Believe me, once you start feeling your feelings and creating a life you are passionate about, you will be experiencing pleasure that no food, no matter how delicious, can compete with. If food has become your sole source of passion, it might be frightening to let it go because it's the only "high" you can imagine today. But let me reassure you that when you let go of compulsive eating, a much wider array of "highs" are immediately available to you. *Every* sensation is intensified when you are connected with your body, so every positive feeling is jacked-up to a higher level.

It is important to get in touch with the activities in your life that bring you the most pleasure, to define for yourself what it is you *really* enjoy doing outside of eating. This may require some trial and error if you have been disconnected from joyous activities for some time, so you've got to once again muscle up and start figuring it out. Being able to divert your attention to those pleasures will serve as empowering alternatives to eating when you are not hungry.

Awareness Opportunity

What are your absolutely favorite things to do?

What is preventing you from incorporating this activity into your life regularly?

Are you doing what you love for a living, and if not, why not?

Old Belief: *Food is the greatest high available to me.*

New Belief: *I am actively creating/living a life that I am passionate about, where pleasure is present in my career, my relationships, my hobbies and my home life.*

I Can Avoid My Feelings Around
an Unpleasant Situation With Food

Avoidance eating often takes place when there are tasks, responsibilities, interactions or goals that are so unappealing or that you dread so much that rather than diving in and getting them over with, you attempt to escape, if even for a brief time, by eating. I know from experience that eating can be a very welcome distraction from digging into a disagreeable chore or responsibility. I have spent entire days mulling, procrastinating and stressing over tasks that, if I had handled them first thing in the morning, I would have been able to enjoy my day unfettered by the tension that precedes a binge.

Today, when I find that I am gravitating towards eating because I am avoiding something, I know the *smartest* thing I can possibly do is to

169

face the avoided task head-on as rapidly as possible. Putting my most unappealing tasks at the very top of my "to do" list each day helps tremendously to make the remainder of my day enjoyable. My neglected task is not occupying valuable space in my head all day long, driving me to eat. Whether it is engaging in a difficult conversation, making a phone call to clean up a conflict or handling basic cleaning chores around the house, I know the sooner I handle it, the better I feel. Freedom from the thoughts about having to do something I dislike feels wonderful. It wipes my psychological slate clean so that I can be fully present for my day. I find that the overwhelming majority of the time procrastinating over the task is *far* worse than digging in and getting it over with. It's the *thinking* about it and my *resistance* to doing it that tends to get me all worked up. Handling the tasks that cause me the most stress as soon as possible has served me powerfully because it takes me to a state of centeredness quickly so I don't have to use food to calm myself.

I have also avoided difficult confrontations for much the same reason. I didn't want to face someone's anger or hurt, and so rather than deal directly, I gorged. I was afraid to lose friendships or look like the bad guy by airing my grievances, so instead I munched. I was afraid to appear selfish, so instead of expressing my needs, I snacked. Sound familiar? Often people with eating issues are sensitive souls who have difficulty with strong emotions, which is why we eat: to avoid our emotions. We're not likely to jump into the lion's den of confrontation if we can help it. But the conflict cannot be reduced if it isn't addressed.

Things are quite different for me now. If I have an issue with someone I

170

care about, I mention it as quickly as possible so I don't have my brain's hard drive full of conflict. Peace is my preference, and I know that I can only attain that if I am willing to be uncomfortable for the short term by meeting with the person I am struggling with and expressing my truth. Remarkably, something great always comes of these "meetings," which inspires me to continue with this self-loving practice of handling conflicts quickly, lovingly and directly.

Awareness Opportunity

What tasks are you putting off that are creating stress in your life?

Does conflict feel like a frightening experience to you?

Who in your life do you avoid conflict with?

Old Belief: *If I eat rather than doing what I need to do, or facing whom I need to face, I will feel better.*

New Belief: *I handle the tasks that cause me the most stress as soon as possible so that I can experience peace as soon as possible,*

The World Is Not a Safe Place

There are many people who share the belief that the world is a bad or dangerous place because of all the heart wrenching things that are taking place–the corruption, the violence, the lack of compassion and understanding. It is a strong belief that is exacerbated by what we watch on television. Violence, self-denigrating behaviors and dysfunction rule the television world, and most of us are watching it all unfold night after night.

Studies show that the average American watches seven hours of television a day and given the popularity of crime and violence-oriented programming, it adds to our untamed mind's fearful nature. When we watch images of violence, whether on the news or on a fictional show, it strengthens our belief that the world is an unsafe place. Even when you know it is "make believe," violence on television can work up your untamed mind, deepening an illusion that things are worse than they are in actuality. This makes us afraid, not only for ourselves, but also for our loved ones. If I watch story after story about murders and rapes and hijackings and stalkers and bitter relationships, I am feeding myself a menu of entertainment that will make me feel more distrustful of others, more fearful of the world I live in. Each violent scene lands somewhere in my psyche and hangs out there. The things we watch and observe are to our mental health as the foods we put into our body are to our physical health. When you are digesting violence, disrespectful behavior and dysfunctional relationships, they weigh you down emotionally. It's therefore no surprise that many people are looking to "protect" themselves by unconsciously adding a barrier of extra weight to guard against having to experience new pains in their future.

While it is evident that there are some incredibly tragic and violent things happening in the world, things that need to be addressed immediately because innocent people are suffering unnecessarily, there are also a significant amount of joyous and inspiring things happening daily. The media doesn't cover those stories with *nearly* as much concentration. It instead focuses on the sensational stories of destruction or violence that garner attention and ratings. If there were a television network devoted to telling stories only about the wonderful things that were happening in the world every day, you would likely feel safer, happier and more optimistic.

Recognizing that there are incredibly wonderful things happening every day on this planet will allow you to experience deeper internal peaceful states. For every death, there is a birth; for every act of violence, there is an act of supreme kindness; for every theft, there is an example of extreme generosity. Residing in fear will only encourage emotional eating and rob you of the many joys that life offers every single day. If you stay locked in the mind-set that the world is negative place, you might not see all the sweetness. You will also miss out on seeing the ultimate truth: that love is ultimately the strongest force on earth.

I (mostly) see the world as an inherently magical and wonderful place, and every event, even the most difficult ones, as opportunities for each of us to evolve, to learn compassion, self-empowerment, unconditional love and the understanding that we are all one. Sometimes I forget this truth, but when I remember it again, I am instantly put back in a more peaceful place. We are, for better or for worse, all in it together, bound by our common humanity. It is our role as residents of this planet to work to change the circumstances that don't serve our global family and to keep a great deal of our focus on the beauty that is available to all of us. This paradigm is such a rich one that it fills us like no chocolate decadence dessert ever could.

Awareness Opportunity

What force do you believe is stronger, love or fear?

What habits do you indulge that contribute to your fears?

What belief about the process of life would allow you to feel more joyous and fearless?

Old Belief: *The world is a scary, unpredictable and unsafe place.*

New Belief: *I am safe within myself, knowing that I have the ability to turn around for the better any challenging situation that comes into my life. Every experience, even the hard ones, are gifts designed to bring me closer with the Divine and with myself.*

There Might Not Be Enough for Me

I once heard it said that we human beings possess two primordial fears: not being enough, and not having enough. I have also found over the years that a common characteristic among compulsive overeaters is that they often have a sense or feeling of lack. They fear that there won't be enough for them—enough attention, enough time, enough love, enough money, enough food. As a result they often go overboard when it comes to their eating habits. They don't feel internal abundance that accompanies self-love, so lack becomes their driving force.

The fear of not having enough often stems from an upbringing where a child did not receive enough love, attention, affection and appreciation. Later in life, as adolescents, teens and adults, we look to fill the void we are feeling with food. Do you ever eat because you are afraid you won't have the chance to eat a particular food again for a while? Do you feel lacking in any or many areas of your life? Most of us do!

However, when you learn to love and appreciate yourself, you will feel a level of abundance that will infiltrate every area of your life. When you connect with the divinity within you, you will know that abundance is your natural state, and that there will *always* be enough for you, in every area of your life. I can often remember eating until I was stuffed to capacity because I knew I would be going on a diet the next day and I was already living in the "lack" of food choices and portions. I'd eat double or even triple portions of foods that I considered special because I was afraid of not having the chance to eat them again. Fear stimulates this mentality, which then stimulates a hoarding behavior (e.g., compulsive eating).

Remind your untamed mind that there will *always* be enough of anything you truly need. Repeating that thought to yourself daily will help quell the fears that drive your emotional appetites. Your outer world of form and experience is a reflection of your inner world of thoughts and feelings. The more you focus on the positive in your life, the more you attract. This is a fact, a universal law, which has been confirmed in the world of physics as well as in daily life. A consciousness of your prosperity will bring about contentment that will gradually eliminate the thought that *there won't be enough for me.*

Take heart in the fact that, like a loving parent, the Divine wants all the best possible for *you*. The Divine isn't like a petulant child who only offers love when you do things perfectly. The Divine is pure love, a love that has no boundaries, no limitations and no expectations. Of course, like a loving parent, the Divine wants us to have true joy in life and, if our actions are not bringing us peace, we will be guided in a different direction by life's experiences and our feelings about our circumstances.

One of the gifts the Divine gives each of us is free will. We are each fully empowered to make all choices for ourselves. This allows us to grow and mature as we identify the choices that are not allowing us to experience life at its best. You are a beautiful expression of the Divine's love. Living in this truth will provide you with a life experience that is fun, exciting, joy-filled, fascinating and peaceful. You can, and deserve to, have it all. Remember that and the floodgates of abundance will continue to swing open. Open your hand and your heart to the goodness that is *always* available to you.

Awareness Opportunity

Do you believe that things happen for a reason?

Do you predominantly think about what you have rather than what you do not have?

Do you feel like you live in fear of lack in any area of your life?

Old Belief: *There might not be enough money, love or food for me in the* *future.*

New Belief: *Abundance on all levels is my natural state and I know that I will always have enough of what I truly need. When I trust this truth, abundance in its many forms flows more easily to me.*

I'm Afraid of Failing

Author, futurist and visionary Buckminster Fuller wrote, "Whatever humans have learned had to be learned as a consequence only of trial and error experience. Humans have learned only through mistakes." While this is undeniably true, our fears of making mistakes and of ultimately failing can prevent us from charging ahead in our lives. For years I used my weight as an excuse for not doing all the things in my life I wanted to do. I was an unwitting *excuse-aholic.* What I discovered about myself, through introspection and coaching, was that I equated losing weight with no longer having an excuse for not going after my dreams. I rarely put one hundred percent into anything I did, and the quality of my life pretty much reflected that average level of fulfillment. So for years I robbed myself of the sense of fulfillment, achievement and empowerment that comes with fully applying oneself, stepping up, focusing deliberately and facing and conquering fears.

For many of us the fear of failing resides at the heart of the excess weight we carry. I didn't figure out until my thirties that failure is only possible if I am not trying at *all,* and that there is *no* shame in trying to make something happen and it not turning out the way I had originally envisioned. I have learned to act boldly and move confidently in the direction of my dreams, and, much to my delight, they are all manifesting, slowly but surely. I had to be willing to take risks and face my fears, but when I did so, whether it was related to my weight-release goals or career goals, I saw my life path unfolding just as I hoped it would. If you want the gold, you've got to be bold!

You might be afraid that if you release the excess weight you are carrying, you will just regain it and your untamed mind will label it yet another failure. You might have already dealt with so much emotional baggage that you don't want to have to deal with the disappointment and frustration on entirely new or different levels. But what if I told you that Thomas Edison tried upwards of one thousand times before the light-bulb became a reality. In reference to how many times he tried to create the light-bulb, he said: "I have not failed. I've just found one thousand ways that won't work." Yowza, what a man! If he had given up hope because he was frustrated or afraid to fail again, we'd live in a very dark world.

The same is true for you. If you keep on trying, even in the face of numerous failures, your light will eventually shine. In truth, the greatest personal success stories are those of people who have had numerous setbacks on their path, but refused to allow themselves to get mired down in feelings of failure. What these individuals had in common is that they didn't allow themselves to feel paralyzed when they made a poor choice, or had an obstacle show up on their path. Instead, they continued to stay focused on their goal, which allowed them to achieve it!

As Franklin Roosevelt once said, "The only thing we have to fear is fear itself." This well-respected leader recognized early on that fear is the greatest block to a life well lived. Remind yourself that it is the loud, nay-saying voice generated by your untamed mind that prevents you from grabbing for the brass ring. Happily, that self-defeating voice can be dramatically reduced once you learn to witness it and shut it down with an internal dialogue that offers a reasonable response for addressing whatever challenge you are facing in a positive and constructive way.

I learned, through direct experience, that if I indulged my fears, I would rarely if ever do *anything* because all my fear would keep me in a small box, reducing my life experience to only the familiar. I have learned to observe myself when I am feeling fearful, and I ask, "Am I in any physical danger?" If the answer is no, then I ignore my untamed mind and I start an inner dialogue where I gently remind myself that my fears very, very rarely materialize. I look back on the years in which I felt paralyzed and overwhelmed with deep appreciation that I am no longer the victim of my phantom fear. The more I overcome my fears, the better I feel. Because I have learned to feel and silence them, I am reaching my goals and achieving my most passionate and heartfelt dreams.

Once you learn to feel the fear and do it anyway, those fears will gradually melt away like ice cubes on a hot stovetop. You cannot fail if you continually take tiny steps towards you goal. Success is the inevitable result of a strong focus!

Awareness Opportunity

Do you think you have ever "failed" at anything?

What did this experience teach you?

Was there anything positive that came of this experience?

Old Belief: *If I fail, I will be even more miserable than I am now.*

New Belief: *I cannot fail if I stay focused on my goals and enjoy the process of creation. It is only a matter of time before all of my dreams are realized if I keep moving ahead by taking consistent steps, no matter how small.*

Awareness Opportunity: The beliefs above represents many of the common beliefs that stand in the way of staying connected with our bodies and our true hungers. Your subconscious mind might have another belief that you know is holding you back from achieving a peaceful relationship with your body. To the best of your ability, articulate what that belief might be.

*****

"Think with your whole body."

–Taisen Deshimaru

Chapter 5

The Ten Keys to Achieving Your Ideal Weight Without Dieting:

How to Eat in Alliance With Your Body

Now that we have covered the *mental* side of releasing weight, there is still another facet of our healing process, the *physical* side. It goes without saying that we can't live without food. We *have* to eat. So, unlike other addictions (think alcohol and drugs), we can't cut out our addictive substance entirely. It is a highly delicate balancing act when you have to moderate yourself around the very thing you are compulsive around. This is why it is vital to have some smart guidelines in place that will support you in finding your balance, ones that will help you stay connected to your body and accurately make the distinction between when you are *physically* hungry from when you are *emotionally* hungry. Essentially, you want to establish a partnership with your body so you can achieve not only your ideal weight, but your ideal health as well.

In this chapter, you will learn the specific keys to make this happen–

without dieting or giving up any of your favorite foods (yahoo!). I call it *Eating in Alliance* with your body because you are eating in *union* with your true physical appetites. An *alliance* is a cooperative relationship based upon an intention to achieve a common goal, in this case achieving your healthiest weight. When you make your body your ally by listening to it and responding to it, eating when you are physically (as opposed to emotionally) hungry and stopping when you are satisfied as opposed to stuffed, *that's* when the excess weight falls away. It is the *natural* way to eat. It is *not* eating to cope with the challenges of life or to distract you from uncomfortable feelings. It *is* eating to fuel your body in a healthy way while you generously treat your taste buds.

You were born with natural and body-connected eating habits that were distorted at some point in your history. With practice, *Eating in Alliance* will allow you to phase out those eating distortions so you can once again eat in synchronicity with your body, listening and responding directly to its signals for hunger and satisfaction. You won't have to count calories, carbohydrates or fat grams and you won't be popping pills or starving yourself. You'll just be returning to an eating style that, at one point in your development, was as natural as smiling when you are in a great mood.

You probably already know a woman who seems to eat whatever she wants without gaining weight. You might think that her good fortune is hereditary; that she hit the genetic jackpot and got a metabolism that allows her to burn through food like a marathon runner with a tapeworm. Although there are some people blessed with a metabolism that works overtime, the more likely scenario is that the people you know who are naturally thin are so because they predominantly eat when they are physically hungry. They *Eat in Alliance* with their bodies rather than eating out of habit or in an effort to avoid feelings. If you observe the people you know who naturally maintain their ideal weight, you will see that they tend to eat the foods they want without censorship, and they don't monitor each and every morsel they put into their mouths in order to stay thin. That confining approach to weight maintenance holds the prison-like energy of dieting, and doing it for a lifetime will rob you of the ease and pleasure that *Eating in Alliance* with your body can provide. People who *Eat in Alliance* tune into their wise bodies so there is no need to weigh food or count calories. How fantastic is that!

While struggling with my compulsive relationship with food, I had quite a few close friends who modeled healthy eating patterns for me, who naturally *Ate in Alliance* with their bodies. They allowed me to see first-hand that it was possible to eat whatever food I craved and still achieve and maintain my natural weight. Having an example of what was possible for me was inspirational. I started to believe that if other women could eat their favorite foods and maintain their ideal weight, I could too. It was a whole new model for me to follow. I recognized that naturally lean people rarely eat for emotional reasons and seldom, if ever, deprive themselves of the food they want. They count on their bodies to inform them, through physical sensations, when it is time to eat and when it is time to stop. And that is what you *too* will learn through following the *Eating in Alliance* keys.

Little babies are *wonderful* models for *Eating in Alliance*. When they are hungry, they usually fuss or cry and, as a result, they get fed. When they feel physically satisfied, they reject the bottle or their mother's breast by pushing it away or by turning their heads to avoid the nipple. Most toddlers and young children eat the same way. Once they feel full, even if they are offered a treat, they usually turn it down. As soon as they are hungry again, they eat something. This is a perfect example of how to *Eat in Alliance*.

Can you remember a time in your life when you thought about food predominantly when your body and not your mind told you to; a time when you ate foods that you loved with uninhibited gusto and never thought about ordering dressing on the side, skinning your chicken dinner or choosing a no-fat dessert; a time when it felt uncomfortable and unappealing to eat when you were not hungry? *Eating in Alliance* with your body will allow you the same freedom once again. You will gradually find that it is virtually *impossible* to eat with the same level of food compulsion that you did before because it feels unnatural and incredibly uncomfortable. You can no longer ignore your body's signals for full. You will instead notice them right away and respond automatically by putting down your fork. After a while it will become a practically effortless practice.

Eating in Alliance requires that you listen to your body the way you listen to your closest friends. Your body knows *exactly* what foods you need at any time to optimize your health and energy levels. It can and will give you explicit cravings for specific foods that provide it with the nutrients it needs to operate optimally. When you pay attention to your body's communications, you will know when it is protein deficient because it will *tell* you by giving you a craving for peanut butter, tofu, meat, fish, beans, poultry or any other food that has high protein content. You'll know when you need more carbohydrates because you'll crave bread, potatoes or another carbohydrate-rich food. When I *truly* listen to my body, I find that I crave much healthier foods. Today I eat lots of highly nutritious foods not because I *have* to, but because I *want* to. I'm still sometimes startled by how easy it has become for me to choose the higher nutrition foods. This does not mean I don't indulge my passion for sugary things. I am still known to have dessert *instead* of dinner now and then. But now that I have reconnected with my true physical appetites, my sugar obsession has diminished and my palate has expanded to include a much larger and healthier array of foods.

In addition to the self-love and body-love practices we've discussed in Chapters 3 and 4, there are *Ten Keys to Eating in Alliance* with your body. The keys will provide you with very specific practices that will allow you to reconnect with your true hunger and achieve your natural weight for good!

So without further ado . . .

Alliance Key #1 – *Enjoy* What You Eat and Give Your Full Attention to Your Meal

One would think that compulsive eaters must really enjoy eating more than the average person since we eat so much and so often. This is not always the case. Those of us dealing with this addiction often feel so guilty about eating that we hardly enjoy our food at all. We often sneak eat or rush anxiously through our meals as though we are in the midst of committing a crime. Our enjoyment of our meal is dramatically diminished because of the shame, tension or regret we feel.

Many times, we are mentally checked-out when eating, completely distracted by our thoughts ("Am I eating the right thing?" "I shouldn't eat too much.'" "Ugh, I'm overeating."), or by a second form of stimulation such as television, reading, surfing the web, driving or talking on the phone. A big part of the reason we overeat is specifically because we are so highly distracted by the *second* activity.

One of the most self-defeating habits I formed at the height of my eating disorder was eating while watching television. Back then I habitually loaded up my plate with goodies and watched my favorite programs while I ate. I loved how it gave me two "highs" simultaneously. It was, however, a very costly habit, one that was responsible for the majority the excess weight I gained. When my focus was on the TV show I was watching rather than the food I was eating, I was only semi-enjoying my meal. Oftentimes it seemed as though the food I had prepared for myself suddenly vanished into thin air. I barely even remembered eating it, which naturally left me feeling dissatisfied and wanting more. Watching television also drowned out my body's signals for "full" and "stop before I explode." So virtually *every* time I ate in front of the television, I ate far more than I was hungry for, but of course, I still felt deprived. That's why I kept making trips back to the kitchen.

I eventually figured out that if I wanted to release excess weight, I *had* to give my food my undivided attention. This is a *big* key, my friend! Allowing any other activity to divert your attention from your food will leave you wanting more, *even* when you are stuffed. Any time you are engaged in *any* other activity while eating, you are sabotaging your ability to stay connected with your body and setting yourself up to overeat. I know how difficult it is to contemplate giving up something that you love to do. Believe me, I was not happy about giving up my double dates with television and food. But I can assure you, even though it may be entertaining to eat in front of the television, or while engaging in any other activity, I promise that it is not *nearly* as fun as living at your ideal weight and being free of an obsession with food. The good news is you can still have both television and food, just not at the same time.

It was uncomfortable at first for me to eat without any distractions, kind of dull. However, nothing diffused my "phantom" or "emotional" appetite faster than focusing solely on my meal. When I was done eating, I was truly satisfied. In fact I got bored with eating much sooner without the companionship of my television to distract me. Dr. David Niven, author of *The 100 Simple Secrets of Happy People*, said, "Television is the creamy filling that distracts us from the substance of our lives." In our case, it distracts us from the full experience of our food. Once you get past your initial resistance to breaking this television/eating habit, it will get much easier, I can guarantee it. This new habit may require you to use a voice with yourself that is gentle…but firm. The loving voice that says, "Yes, of course you can watch television, but I'm going to encourage you to eat your entire meal *first* so that you can stay connected with your body. I know how much you want to achieve your natural weight and I'm going to support you in doing just that." You can have your cake, and you can eat it too, just not while you are watching television!

If you are living with someone, I suggest asking for their support to help you break the TV distraction habit. *Everyone* can benefit from devoting their full attention to their meals and their partnership will make it easier to break the double distraction pattern.

Focusing exclusively on your food will not only help you to hear your body's signal for "stop," but it will also help you to enjoy your food *far* more. If you genuinely enjoy your food, you are less likely to overeat because you will feel satisfied with less. And I do mean "enjoy" in the strongest sense of the word. When I eat, I am passionate about each bite I take. Whereas before I barely tasted the food after the first few bites, now I revel in my meals, savoring each bite with great gusto and appreciation. Some of my friends laugh at my unbridled enthusiasm for food and the obvious pleasure I display when I eat. I can't recall enjoying my food *nearly* as much when I was eating compulsively.

Remind yourself, before you put anything in your mouth, that the most *important* thing you can do in that moment is to enjoy what you eat. In the beginning, it might help if you act as if you are in a play and your role is to be a character who is enjoying a meal– to the extreme. Allow little moans of palate pleasure to escape your lips as you eat something delicious. Let your senses take in every detail of what you are eating, the texture, the smell, the taste(s) and even the color of your food.

If you consistently perform this one practice, you will steadily see shifts in your urges to binge. As it did in my case, something inside of you will relax around food. The simple act of focusing on your meal will help you to feel centered as you eat rather than anxious or numb. When you enjoy what you eat and stay present to your food, you grant yourself an internal permission that will feel liberating. You will no longer feel restricted, guilty and rushed, so there is no reason to rebel and eat past your true hungers. If you don't think you can commit to eating all your meals without distractions, start by focusing on eating one meal a day without them. Once you realize the direct relationship between distraction-free eating and releasing excess weight, you'll ease into this way of eating consistently because you will be totally inspired by the weight release that accompanies it.

Eating a delicious meal is one of life's greatest pleasures, one that you can experience each and every day. Remind yourself how important it is to enjoy your food before each and every bite you put in your mouth and see what happens!

Alliance Key #2 – Start Eating When You Are Physically Hungry

Most of us gain excess weight because *we eat when we are not physically hungry*. Think of your stomach like you would a gasoline tank. Would you put gasoline into your tank if you already had a full tank? Or half a tank? Or even a quarter of a tank? Unless you were going on a long trip, you would probably wait until your tank was low on gas, or even close to empty, before stopping at the station to fill it up. It is smart to fuel your body in a similar fashion. You want to fill it up when it is empty, or close to empty, not when it already has ample fuel (food).

Below is a "Hunger Range" that will help you become more aware of when you are *Eating* in or out of *Alliance* with your body. It will support you in recognizing when you are putting in excess fuel. To give you a real handle on hunger ranges, I have included stages that range from "Super Hungry" to "Gorged" with varying degrees of satiation in between. *The key to releasing excess weight is to begin to eat at a Stage Zero to One and to stop eating when you reach a Stage Five to Six.*

Stage Zero = *Super Hungry.* You have unmistakable and sometimes uncomfortable signs of hunger, which might include lightheadedness, nausea and/or hunger pains, a gurgling and empty feeling in your stomach and possibly mood swings. Others experience a "high" when they are hungry.

Stage One = *Hungry.* Your body wants to eat now, and it lets you know by a physical sensation, such as rumbling or an empty feeling in your stomach and some of the other sensations listed above. For some, this stage is accompanied by a "light" feeling.

Stage Two = *Semi-Hungry.* You are a few bites into the meal and the strong hunger cues are gone, but you are not yet close to satisfied.

Stage Three = *Neutral.* Middle of the meal feeling, you feel as if you'd still like some additional food.

Stage Four = *Semi-Satiated.* You are now just a few bites from satisfied.

Stage Five = *Satisfied.* Your body is sending you no hunger cues. You feel perfectly comfortable, like you have had the ideal amount of food.

Stage Six = *Full.* You've taken a few extra bites beyond satisfied and are not getting any hunger signals at all.

Stage Seven = *Very Full.* You've had a full extra portion and know you've gone beyond your true hunger. You are experiencing mild physical discomfort.

Stage Eight = *Stuffed.* You're not hungry at all, but you're eating anyway. Your body is telling you to stop through an overly full feeling in your belly. Your body is giving you a variety of signs of discomfort.

Stage Nine = *Bursting.* You continue to feed your body even though it is telling you "No" through your great discomfort.

Stage Ten = *Gorged.* You couldn't eat another bite without getting sick. Your body is overwhelmed and exhausted and telling you so through intense pain or discomfort.

If you are eating between Stages Seven and Ten, you are eating well beyond your true physical hunger. *This* is where you will gain excess weight. Consistently eating between a Stage Zero to One and stopping at a Five or Six is where you will release any excess weight you carry. It is that simple.

I cannot stress strongly enough the importance of waiting to eat until you are absolutely certain that you feel physically hungry (Stage Zero or One). Why? Because waiting until you get the clear cues to eat is imperative to staying connected to your body. If you do not wait until you hit a Stage Zero/One to eat, it will be *much* more difficult to assess when you hit Stage Five/Six.

Start to pay attention to how often you begin to eat at a Stage Two or Three and how much easier it is to lose track and go beyond a Stage Five/Six when you start eating before you get the clear signals for hunger.

Many individuals who have a compulsive relationship with food might find that they initially have some difficulty identifying what true hunger feels like. They have been disconnected from their true appetites for so long that they literally forget what it feels like to be hungry. Each body experiences hunger differently, and identifying your body's particular cues for hunger is the key. Allow yourself to experiment. Put larger periods of time between your meals than usual and the hunger cues will become quite obvious.

There are a few general hunger communication cues that you might already know. When physical hunger shows, you might feel a hollow or empty sensation in your stomach, or feel it rumbling in anticipation of a meal. You might feel a little light-headed or even hyper and anxious. Some people get a light feeling that they enjoy. Some individuals feel irritable and cranky when they are hungry, others slightly nauseated, and some report feeling a slight headache and/or a drop off in their ability to concentrate. These are all ways that your body communicates to you its needs for nourishment. True hunger will be virtually unmistakable for you once you get back into sync with your body.

If you want to be *sure* what you are experiencing is a physical rather than an emotional hunger, there are a few clues that will help you to differentiate. First you have to slow down so you can truly connect with your body. Sit down in a comfortable chair and take three (or more) deep breaths in through your nose and out through your mouth. Expand your belly like a beach ball with your in-breath, and on your out-breath, allow it to deflate entirely. This simple breathing technique will center and relax you, allowing you greater access to your body's wisdom. As you breathe, ask yourself and your body what hunger stage it is experiencing.

Another powerful technique I use to see if I am legitimately physically hungry is to drink a glass of water. If you can feel it coursing through your body, especially through your throat and upper chest area, it is a clear sign that it is time to eat.

It may take a little time to learn how to wait until you are at a Stage Zero to One to eat. At first, it may feel very uncomfortable. Your untamed mind may be goading you to eat to block out the feelings of discomfort. So what do you do (other than eat) to nurture yourself if you're feeling emotionally hungry? The first step is to pinpoint the *feeling* of discomfort that is making you want to eat (stress, fear, boredom). Next, try to identify what, specifically, is driving the feeling (negative thoughts about yourself, your body or life in general, work stress, conflict within a relationship). And finally, you need to find positive ways to nurture and calm yourself as an alternative to eating (see Chapter 8).

To get myself calm and past the urge to eat when I was not hungry, I used to speak gently to that part of myself that was confused, frightened and nervous (my inner child) in the most gentle, patient, strong and compassionate way I was able. I would use the tender and sweet voice of the most loving mother images I could imagine. By now you have an understanding that your eating compulsions are not about the food; many of them are related to your inner child's need for some form of nurturing and understanding. That part of you that was hurt early in life and is attempting to take care of yourself with food. In that respect, when you are tempted to eat when you are not hungry, it is important to get in touch with your inner child and find out what it is she *really* wants. Reassure your inner child that "Yes, *of course* you can have that food, but let's wait until you are truly hungry because that's when you will feel best eating." Remind yourself that you can have any food you want, as soon as you are truly hungry. Being able to breathe through the urge to eat when you are not hungry will provide you with feelings of freedom and great personal strength.

An internal dialogue with your inner child is one of the most efficient ways I have ever found to overcome a binge. Loving and nurturing the child-like part of yourself that hungers for attention, calm and understanding will deepen your relationship with yourself and ultimately create the peace of mind you are looking for through food. It adds to the trust that you are building in your own sacred inner sanctuary.

For many compulsive overeaters, their inner child runs the show. She is the part of you that forgets that when she eats too much, she'll get a stomachache or feel physically uncomfortable in some other way. When your inner child is always in charge, she will consistently make short-term choices (e.g., eating when you are not hungry) because she has a difficult time delaying gratification. She doesn't consider the future or the ramifications of her choices. For her, it is *all* about the moment. Your inner child can't fully grasp the fact that short-term choices lead to long-term grief where eating is concerned. This is why it's important to coach your inner child, gently and firmly, through the non-hunger related urges to eat. Gently guide your inner child by reminding her of the feeling she gets when she overeats (sluggish, depressed, weak) and that your intention is to guide her to eat in response to her body's needs so she can feel empowered all the time.

Once you remind her that she can have any food she loves if she is *truly* hungry, it will calm her (you) down. When you remind her in the heat of the urge to binge that eating more than she is physically hungry for has negative ramifications, her demands for food will lessen dramatically, as will your urges to binge. Like any child, your inner child thrives on healthy boundaries. It will feel good to her when you put a healthy boundary in place, such as waiting until you are at a Stage Zero/One to

195

eat. It might take a little time to get comfortable communicating with yourself in this intimate, loving mother/daughter fashion, but again, it works, so work it!

Frequently Remind Yourself of the Benefits

Waiting until you are at a Stage Zero/One to eat has many benefits, in addition to weight release. One of my favorites is the fact that food tastes dramatically more flavorful at a Zero/One than when you are eating between a Seven and Ten. Why? Because your taste buds *intensify* when you are really hungry. Flavors get stronger, fuller and more discernable. It is yet another way that your marvelous body lets you know that you are *Eating in Alliance* with your body. After all, the purpose of eating is not *only* to energize and nourish your body, but also to experience *tremendous* pleasure.

Once you get into the rhythm of eating when you are hungry, you will relish the heightened intensity of your food's flavor. If you have the additional motivation of knowing how much better your meal will taste, it can make it easier to wait to eat until you hit a Stage Zero/One. Let your taste buds work in your favor. Here's another tidbit of information that is helpful. After your body is hitting the "satisfied" stage, your taste buds start getting a little "bored." So when the food you are eating starts tasting a little, or a lot "less" delicious, it is another signal that you are approaching a Stage Five and it's time to slow down or stop altogether.

Yet another positive aspect of waiting until you are at a Stage Zero/One is that it gives your stomach time to fully digest your food, which helps your body operate at its highest potential. This translates to optimum health because your body is not being overtaxed. Conversely, if your body is working non-stop to digest food because you are *constantly* eating, it is easy to see how your body can get overwhelmed and exhausted.

Each time you move past the urge to eat when you are not hungry, take a moment to acknowledge and appreciate yourself. Be as effusive as you can in your self-adoration. Out loud or in your head say to yourself, "Fantastic!" "You did it!" "I'm so proud of you!" "Great job!" "I know it was difficult, and I'm impressed with how you worked through it." Coach yourself with great enthusiasm, and you will be even *more* inspired to breathe through your difficult feelings the next time an emotional urge to eat shows up. We all respond well to positive affirmations, whether they come from ourselves or someone else. This is not the time to be shy or self-conscious. No one has to be aware of your outrageously loving inner dialogue but you. Keep in mind as incentive the fact that the more your coach yourself lovingly, the faster you will be able to breathe through the urge to overeat.

Repetition is key to creating a new habit. There's no way around it. Every time you practice waiting until you are hungry to eat, you are building a new path in your psyche that you will eventually revert to naturally. Over and over again, flex your muscle of emotional strength by checking in with your body, breathing, positively coaching yourself and waiting until you are a Stage Zero/One to eat, and you can be absolutely certain that you will gain mastery over your emotional appetites.

Alliance Key #3 - Eat Until You Are Satisfied

Returning to the gas tank analogy, if you continue to put gasoline in your tank when it already registers full, it is going to start to overflow. It's the same with your body. If you are putting food in your body when you are not physically hungry, the excess food has to go somewhere, and predictably, it shows up as excess weight.

You might be surprised at how little food it takes to feel satisfied. Your stomach is approximately the size of your fist (surprising but true). While it is true that your stomach can expand dramatically, it operates most efficiently when the portions align with your true hunger. Take a moment and curl your hand into a fist and hold it out in front of you so you can get a better idea about the size of your stomach. This will support you in building an understanding of the *approximate* amount of food it will take for you to begin to experience a sense of satiation. Keep in mind that I'm referring to a fist-sized portion of food *once it's been properly chewed.*

As your body is unique, you will have to determine for yourself what portion sizes generally work for you. I found that starting out with a small portion and building up was helpful for me. I started out with a small bowl full of food as opposed to the traditional dinner plate I had always used. Through experimentation I found that a medium-sized bowl of food was generally the amount required by my body to hit a Stage Five/Six, though my portions would fluctuate in tandem with the intensity of my workout schedule and how much water I drank.

For some it will take a bowl full of food to feel satisfied, for others a full dinner plate. Honor your own physical appetites and what feels right to you. Start with a bowl full, and then gradually add to that portion size until you find the average portion you require to feel satiated. Start with a bowl or soup cup that is about 5 inches across the top. Once you get clear on how much is required to reach a Stage Five/Six, serve yourself that amount on average at mealtimes and be fully present to each and every delicious bite.

Most people who are *Eating in Alliance* find that smaller portions satisfy them completely once they reconnect with their true appetites. Eating meals that are smaller, and completely gratifying to your taste buds, means you'll probably be eating more frequently throughout the day *and* you will be fully satiated after each meal.

If you happen to eat beyond a Stage Five/Six and feel overly full, don't panic or get angry with yourself. This might throw you into a full-blown binge. To get back on track, just wait until you are at a Stage Zero/One to eat again. It's that simple. If you ate to a Stage Seven last night at your favorite restaurant, you might not hit a Stage Zero/One until 10:30 the next morning or perhaps even later. If you wait until then to eat, that's *all* you have to do to get back in sync with your body! Your body will give you hunger cues to let you know when it is ready for more food. Remember, just because it is morning doesn't mean that it is time for breakfast. Let your body be your barometer.

Alliance Key #4 - Choose Foods You *Really* Love

As a child I lived in San Francisco, and my closest girlfriend, Helen, lived directly across the street. I *loved* going over to her house to play because there was always an abundance of candy, chips and snacks. Helen's incredibly sweet mother, Dawn, loved to indulge both of us with treats. She was English, and afternoon tea was a ritual she observed frequently. She had lovely tea parties for Helen and me in her upstairs sunroom, serving us hot English breakfast tea with plenty of cream and sugar, accompanied by cookies, tiny cakes and candy. It was heavenly! Going to Helen's house and being indulged by her mom was a dream come true for a little girl who craved sugar.

At my house, in my mother's sincere effort to make sure that my three sisters and I stayed healthy, our food and snack choices were quite limited. There was *rarely* an abundance of candy or junk food on hand, and eating between meals was usually a no-no. Partially because sugar was limited at my home, my obsession with it intensified.

In contrast, Helen was allowed to eat whatever and whenever she wanted. It always surprised me that even though she could have anything she wanted to eat, she habitually gravitated to the healthiest foods. I can remember her eating bell peppers and apples, even though Ding-Dongs, Oreos and Otter Pops were always available to her. Don't get me wrong, if she wanted a Ding-Dong, or even two, she had them. However, because she usually waited until she was hungry to eat and paid attention to her body's cravings, she naturally gravitated to healthier food choices overall. Helen is a great example of *Eating in Alliance*. She has always *allowed* herself the choice of any food she wants, and her relationship with it is healthy and balanced.

As I learned later in life, *restricting* your food choices is a high-speed way guaranteed to ignite a compulsion. Start limiting yourself and you are buying a ticket for the express train to compulsion town. That is why it is so very important to equalize every food in your mind. By this I mean letting go of the "good food"/"bad food" paradigm. This means that spinach salad, peach cobbler, artichokes, pesto pasta and chocolate chunk ice cream are all held as "good foods." Yes, you heard me right.

The fact is that *any* food choice can be "good." It is only when that food is eaten to excess that it becomes unhealthy. If you lock into the perception that there are "bad foods," you set yourself up to feel good only when you are eating foods that fit into a restricted mind-set. Labeling foods as "bad" creates the dieter mindset that got you *Eating out of Alliance* with your body in the first place. All foods, even the ones with limited nutritional value, are absolutely fine in moderation, and your ability to eat them in balance will only happen once you stop denying yourself the option to eat them!

If you have a difficult time seeing a food with limited or no nutritional value as "good," see it as "neutral." This will lessen your compulsive eating tendencies because you won't be feeling the guilt that often accompanies thinking you have been or eaten something "bad." While I agree that it is important to have a sound knowledge of nutrition and to eat the healthiest foods possible, for compulsive overeaters, there must *first* be a stage in which they allow themselves any and all foods in order to first move beyond the compulsion. (The exception to this rule is for individuals who have food allergies and/or a medical condition such as diabetes. If you have either of these conditions, you may have to tailor your food choices to honor your body's current condition. Please consult with your doctor if you have any questions along these lines.)

It is important and downright *smart* to eat foods that you love and crave! That's where the obsession with food starts to go away! It is *not* okay to eat something you *don't* like just because you think it is healthier or has fewer calories. That just mimics that "make ya crazy" dieter's mentality. The wonderful news is that your fixation with less nutritious foods will dwindle if you allow yourself complete and *total* access to them. In his best-selling book, *Diets Don't Work*, author Bob Schwartz discusses a food study that was conducted in an orphanage. The children in the study were told that they could choose any food they wanted to eat for thirty days. They were offered a smorgasbord of choices, including both high– and low–nutrient foods. From spinach to chocolate, they had it all. There was one little boy who, on the first day of the study, had Cracker Jacks for breakfast, lunch and dinner. At first, the researchers found this quite funny and cute but with each day, as he continued to load his plate with the sugary popcorn, they grew increasingly concerned about his well-being. Fortunately they didn't have to worry. After he had completely indulged his obsession with Cracker Jacks, he went on to start eating foods with far greater nutritional content. At the end of the thirty-day period, the doctors added up everything the little fellow had eaten and it turned out to be a balanced diet! His body started to crave high-nutrition foods to balance out all the caramel corn he had eaten. Without any guidance whatsoever from the adults, this little boy connected with his body, which eventually guided him to more nutritious foods. Rejoice, my friend, because your body will do the same for you once you reconnect with its communications.

Again, although there are many theories as to the healthiest ways to eat, no one can assess the foods that compliment your health and energy levels as accurately as you, and your brilliant body, can. The most important factor to consider as you make your food selection is how those foods make your body *feel*. If you feel awful after eating a tomato, you know that it is not the best choice for your individual body, even if tomatoes are very nutritious.

Have a blast experimenting with different foods. Go ahead, be celebratory as you embark on this new relationship with food and your body. Be sure to eat all of your favorites, and try things you haven't tasted before! Honor all of your cravings and remind yourself that by allowing yourself to eat what you truly *love*, you'll feel truly *satiated*. Total freedom around all foods will *help* to break you of a neurotic preoccupation with them. You'll be far more relaxed in your eating habits if you allow yourself the full spectrum of foods!

When I first started to *Eat in Alliance* with my body, I slowly began to allow myself a lot of the foods that I had previously considered off-limits. It was scary, I'll admit. I didn't yet trust myself around food. But I gradually started to trust the "all foods are equal" rule. I chose *exactly* what I wanted and sometimes that meant eating ice cream for breakfast and dinner (I'm not joking). Yet, I noticed I was *still* releasing excess weight even though I was eating the foods that I had previously considered fattening and "bad." This was because I was eating between a Stage Zero and a Stage Six the great majority of the time. Eventually, as I re-connected with my body on a far more intimate level, my urges for sugar diminished substantially and I now hunger for foods that are delicious and also packed with nutritional value because they make me feel so energetic. I crave salads, fruits, nuts and vegetables with as much relish as I once had for Sugar Babies and Pepperidge Farm cookies (those tasty treats rock!).

The more connected you are with your body, the less you will crave foods that drain you of energy. That is partially because feeling good in your body becomes even more pleasurable than the best "food high" you have ever experienced. You don't have to take my word for it. Try it yourself!

When you first start this process you may find, like I did, that you too are eating lots of foods you previously considered "off-limits." This is common (and fun, I might add) and a perfectly acceptable adjustment period to a new way of relating to food…and it will not last forever. If you want pancakes for dinner, go for it. If you are dying for a piece of berry pie in the morning, knock yourself out! And enjoy it *massively* if you want to lessen your obsession with it.

As you are gaining self-awareness in the ways I've described, become more aware of how your appetite varies when you are faced with a shift in your physical or emotional state. I have far more cravings for sugar during my menstrual cycle or when I am under extra pressure in my personal life or my career. During those times, I am exceptionally gentle with myself and am even more attentive to the signals my body is sending to me in terms of cravings. I know beyond a shadow of a doubt that when I am craving sugary food with a greater intensity, I need to pay attention to what may be happening in my life that needs to be accepted, changed or even eliminated. During those times I will not judge myself for my high-sugar food choice, but will wait until I am hungry to eat my dessert. Remember, it is not about *what* you eat, but *when* and *how much* you eat that ultimately dictates your weight. This is a lifetime program and denying yourself any of your favorite foods is not necessary…or effective!

When you are starting out, if you are not sure about what specific food you want for breakfast, lunch or dinner, conduct your own little "taste test." Experiment with the different tastes by visualizing eating the food of your choice before you take even one bite, doing your best to conjure up the texture, the temperature, the taste, the smell and the flavor of the food. Run the experience of the specific food through your mouth so you can assess your potential satisfaction with your choice upfront. And while you are at it, question yourself thoroughly. Are you craving something hot or cold, something sweet or salty, something crunchy or smooth? You can eat *anything* you want as long as you are hungry. Joy Colangelo, my friend and the author of *Embodied Wisdom*, told me that before she eats anything, she asks herself, "Is this a 'yes' for my body?" Start to tap into what your yes foods are and make sure you have an abundance of them in your kitchen. When you slow down and listen to your body's guidance, you'll be in the care of the most brilliant nutritionist on the planet.

Alliance Key #5 - Eat as Slowly as Possible

Learning to eat slowly will be a key factor in your ability to release excess weight and keep it off. When I was at the height of my food compulsion, I ate so quickly that I seldom noticed the textures, smells or flavors of my meals. If you throw in the multitasking I used to do while I was compulsively eating, it is clear why I rarely, if ever, felt satisfied with a meal.

When I eat slowly and consciously, however, making sure to enjoy every little bite, I feel satisfied much sooner *and* I know with greater clarity when I reach a Stage Five/Six. Eating at a leisurely pace allows me to fully indulge myself in the experience of the textures, flavors, scents and even the visual appeal of the food. I *love* to eat, and it has become a far more enjoyable experience because I no longer feel guilty after my meals. In fact, I feel really excited to eat most of the time. Eating is one of life's greatest pleasures, which is why it is so important to linger over meals, and draw them out, like a wonderful conversation.

Here's a wonderful practice: Begin to deliberately stretch out your meals for as long as possible. The goal of this is to pay as much attention to your food as you can. Remember to remind yourself before a meal: The slower I eat this food, the more satisfied I will feel. The more satiated you feel, the less likely you will be to overeat or even binge. If you want to have a little fun with this practice, set a timer and start to challenge yourself to prolong your meals as long as you can. Make it an empowering game.

Yet another benefit of eating slowly is that it enhances your digestion process! Good digestion might not be at the top of your current priority list, but anyone who has experienced the discomfort of overeating can attest to the ramifications of eating too quickly. Stomachaches, indigestion, nausea, I remember how awful I felt after a rushed refrigerator raid. Eating slowly has eliminated those conditions from my life entirely.

When I was first learning to *Eat in Alliance*, I developed a few tricks to help me slow down during my meals. One of them was eating with my non-dominant hand. Although I was born right-handed, I would intentionally eat with my left hand when I caught myself eating compulsively. This was a great "wake up" technique simply because the awkwardness of eating with my left hand forced me to eat more slowly. It turned out to be an effective tool. I also learned to put my fork down after every single bite and to chew my food *very, very* well. When you are first beginning, you can exaggerate this by making it a goal to see how many times you can chew your food before swallowing.

Challenge yourself to *exaggerate* your slow eating. Go as far as pretending you are eating in slow motion. Make it a production or performance that you regularly engage in. You may feel a little silly at first, but who the heck cares! The benefits will quickly outweigh any awkwardness you may feel. Practice daily. The more you eat slowly, the faster it will become an ingrained habit that you won't even have to think about!

Alliance Key #6 – Take Three Conscious Breaths Before Eating Anything

One of the defining qualities of my compulsive eating style was that I reached for food so habitually, so automatically and rapidly, that there was rarely a moment of contemplation between the impulse to eat and the act of eating. I can own the fact that I was a world-class speed eater. A feeling (usually an uncomfortable one) triggered a non-hunger related urge to eat, and I headed right for the refrigerator, not stopping for a *minute* to think about the ramifications of my choice. I had to train myself away from this knee-jerk reaction, to stop before I was left looking at the very bottom of ice cream carton.

So how *do* you stop? Or at least slow yourself down?

One of *the* most effective tools I have found is the simple act of *deep breathing*. Taking three conscious breaths *before you eat anything* will help center and relax you so that you can then make a far more deliberate and controlled choice to eat or not to eat. Slow breathing will slow you down and help to calm the feelings that are driving your non-hunger related urges to eat. From this composed, more centered place, it will also be easier to follow through with the other *Eating in Alliance* keys. Oftentimes I am just a few breaths away from transcending a binge urge. When stressed you will involuntarily stop breathing for spurts of time, which will make you feel even more tense! Deep breathing will unquestioningly break that tension-inducing habit.

My conscious breath, more so than any other factor, provides me with the opportunity to pause and evaluate my choices about eating. By choices I mean not just *if* I will eat, but *what* I will eat if I choose to. Breathing deeply has stopped me from bingeing many, many times because it awakened me to the moment, allowing me to remember that *nothing* tastes as good as being connected to my body and living at my natural weight.

So how *do* you breathe consciously? Don't you already breathe? Yes of course, but most of us commonly breathe in a shallow fashion from the upper chest rather than from the depths of our lungs. It works this way. When we are tense our breathing shifts automatically to our upper chest to prepare us to either defend ourselves or to flee the scene. It is as though we are *on the ready* preparing for some form of an altercation all the time. This shallow breathing pattern is affiliated with the "fight or flight" response of our earliest genetics. I consider this shallow breathing somewhat of a leftover from our early genetics because fleeing and fighting aren't nearly as commonplace today as they were with our ancestors, who were dealing with sabre toothed tigers rather than traffic jams. But the main point here is that when you breathe in a shallow fashion it ends up creating a feeling of stress that can *contribute* to your compulsive eating tendencies.

When you breathe deeply, on the other hand, you naturally loosen up. Conscious breathing requires that you pay close attention to your breath as you breathe deeply, from your belly. When you breathe into your belly, you are *automatically* initiating a relaxation response that will allow you to melt into a calmer state. It is the ultimate natural tranquilizer! Here's another great body fact: When you breathe, you are nourishing your body! You breathe oxygen into your lungs, which then travels through your bloodstream to nourish your cells. How does it feel to know that simply by taking a deep breath you are doing something really wonderful for yourself? I think it feels *fantastic* if I do say so myself!

If you want to see how to breathe properly, take a peek at a tiny baby when they are sleeping. Babies offer outrageously cute examples of natural and healthy breathing. If you watch a baby sleep, you will notice that they breathe *slowly* and *deeply* into their bellies. A baby will inhale through its nose until its tummy fills out like a little beach ball and then will exhale through its nose and/or mouth. Practice putting your hands on your abdomen and extending your stomach in concert with your inhaled breath, and emptying it in concert with the exhale. I invite you to try it several times now so that you will remember it for future reference. This breathing pattern will ensure that the nourishment that the breath provides will infiltrate your entire body. You can exhale through your mouth, but it is best to do it through your nose. Think of your nose is your "air hole" and your mouth your "food hole" (crass but accurate).

Like your thought-observation practice, start to observe how you *breathe* throughout the day. Do you frequently hold your breath? Do you

210

generally breathe deeply or in a shallow fashion? Do you tend to breathe from your chest or your belly? When you slow down long enough to get in touch with your breath and you retrain yourself to breathe more deeply consistently, you will access a level of peace that is *priceless*.

I could *easily* dedicate an entire chapter to the benefits of healthy breathing. Gay Hendrick's book, *Conscious Breathing*, changed my breathing habits for good, and I recommend it with *massive* enthusiasm. Breathing is the first thing you do when you are born and the last thing you do before you die! It's the connecting force to life. Now *that's* a big deal!

Did you know that humans breathe, on average, 20,000 times a day? It makes *total* sense that even a slight shift for the better in something that you do that many times a day can make a huge difference. Breathing deeply can reduce your stress levels and provide you with immediate pleasure, a natural high that becomes a healthy substitute for food as a form of self-nurturing. Breathing well is tantamount to chilling out!

The fact is that it is much easier to change an old habit if you have a new and healthy one to replace it. Conscious breathing can be that replacement behavior that creates the pleasurable high or calming factor you were seeking through food. Your breath is always available to you, always reliable, has zero calories and it doesn't cost a cent! Start practicing this breathing technique as often as possible, even when you *aren't* tempted to binge, so that it becomes second nature. That way you can defer to it immediately when you are in particularly stressful moments.

Sometimes if I feel I *really* need to chill having worked myself up by paying too much attention to my untamed mind, I hold my breath as long as I can and then I take a huge inhale of oxygen once I let go. I do this a few times and it has a hugely calming effect on me. I have a strong tendency to hold my breath when I am tense so when I flood my body with the nourishment of a *really* deep breath, I am considerably soothed. I have put signs in strategic places at my house that say "breathe" to remind me to relax myself throughout the day. I have one on my phone, one on my refrigerator and one on my computer. My stress levels have never been lower, and I know that breathing is in large part responsible for this happy fact. An oxygen cocktail in the form of deep breathing can provide you with a natural high, a feeling of euphoria without the hangover. Now that's the kind of party we all want to be invited to!

Alliance Key # 7 -Eat Only When Seated

This *Eating in Alliance* key ties into Key #1 (Enjoy Your Food) and is a vital part of your process. Why? Because if you are standing while eating it suggests that you are in a rush, which means you are depriving yourself of the full experience of your food. Like eating with distractions, if you are eating while standing, you will end up feeling unsatisfied.

This is especially true for those of us that have a tendency to graze at the refrigerator or cupboards without sitting down to really enjoy a meal. I know that for me there was often a guilt factor involved when I was standing and eating straight from the refrigerator, almost like I felt I *shouldn't* really be eating, but I couldn't help myself, so was rushing through it.

Eating while seated is a powerful practice. You might be surprised at how much this one key will increase the amount you enjoy your food and decrease the amount of food you eat. Commit to yourself that you will sit down before you eat or drink anything, *even if it is on the floor in front of the refrigerator or pantry.* (I did this many times during my healing process.) When I caught myself sitting on my kitchen floor, it was a little wake-up call that often allowed me to stop eating compulsively much sooner. I was not fully aware of how much my standing and eating habit contributed to my binges until I stopped doing it. Following this key woke me up to a pattern that was sabotaging me for years, and I'm happy to say that it can do the same for you!

Slowing down to enjoy your meal as you sit at your dinner table is crucial because you will be able to recognize with greater accuracy when you feel satiated (Stages Five/Six). When you are eating out of the refrigerator it is difficult to keep track if you have eaten a fist-sized portion of food or a feast-sized portion. If you find yourself standing and eating, gently coach yourself by saying out loud, "I am eating while standing and I'm going to stop now." This single observation, once vocalized, may be all that it takes to get you to either sit down and be present to your meal or maybe even make the choice to turn away from food in the moment.

Alliance Key #8 - Stay Well-Hydrated and Drink at Least One Glass of Water With Each Meal

There was a time in my life when my plants got more water than I did. No joke. I actually disliked water, finding it an exceptionally dull alternative to the many other flavors available to me. It felt like a burden to drink it, so I rarely did. Which is why I was always dehydrated. Apparently studies show that seventy-five percent of my fellow-Americans are too.

Drinking water is one of the *most* important things you can do for your health and one of the most proactive things you can do to release excess weight and maintain that loss. If you are chronically dehydrated, you are highly likely to mistake thirst for hunger and reach for food when what you *really* need to feel satiated and calm is a glass of water. Think of it this way. Your body orders a drink of water and you give it a sandwich or a cookie instead. If you ordered one thing in a restaurant and were given something completely different, you'd probably be annoyed, and I imagine that's how your body feels under similar circumstances. Be aware of your thirst signals!

Once you get in the habit of drinking water regularly, you'll realize how often you used to reach for food when you were actually just *thirsty*! Whenever I am unsure as to whether I am hungry or thirsty, I start by having a tall glass of water. My body then lets me know, through a feeling of satisfaction that water was what was called for. After a full glass of water, I am not *nearly* as tempted to binge and I have more energy to boot. You will find that when you are properly hydrated, your urges to overeat will diminish substantially.

Not only will drinking water help you achieve your natural weight, it will also positively increase other aspects of your health. Water is second only to air in terms of your survival, even before food. Although you can go for weeks without eating, the maximum time you can survive without water is only a few days. Every cell in your body benefits from a water boost. Rolf Faste, a water expert and professor at Stanford University, explained to me that the more water you drink, the greater the oxygen levels in your cells. This in turn supports good health and high energy levels. In addition, the National Institutes of Health published a study that showed that a lack of water was determined to be the number *one* trigger for daytime fatigue. I can remember a time when I felt really tired in the afternoon and so I would snack heavily, looking to food to pick up my energy level. Now I drink a glass of water as a healthy alternative, and (finally) it doesn't feel like it is an effort. And we all know that water helps to keep your skin looking great. The bonuses are endless!

So how much water is enough? Just as different people have different nutritional needs, each body will have a unique requirement for water, based upon a number of factors including height, weight and activity levels. If you rarely drink water and do not like it very much (yet), start by introducing four glasses of water a day and add to your intake depending on your level of activity and thirst. A day at the beach will require more water than a day in the office. If you are a long-distance runner, you may need more than eight glasses a day. Remember, it is better to err on the side of too much water than too little. It is *never* appropriate, however, to overstuff your body with anything, solid or liquid. You also might not want to spend your entire day in the bathroom, so play with the water doses and see what works for you.

Many of us are so out of touch with our bodies that, like our signals for hunger, we don't notice the signals for extreme thirst. In fact, if you are thirsty, you are already dehydrated! Your thirst mechanisms only kick in when you are already hitting the dehydrated stages. And it takes about two hours for the water you drink to have an effect on your body's hydration level. You have to stay ahead of the thirsty sensation to be properly hydrated! Ideally you don't want to get a dehydrated state simply because it overtaxes your body. That's why regularly drinking water throughout the day and with each meal is so important, even if you don't feel thirsty.

I have a tall, green-tinted drinking glass on which I have written the words health, love, beauty, abundance and peace in gold permanent pen so that every time I take a drink of water from it, I feel like I am doing something really self-loving. It makes me feel more inspired to drink water when I make a ritual out of drinking from this particular glass. As I drink, I think of all the healthy things the water is doing for my body and it becomes much easier to silence the part of my untamed mind that is trying to get me to eat a candy bar instead. I also have a water bottle in my car at all times so that I can drink throughout the day. Water changed my relationship to my body, and it will do the same for you. I'll drink to that!

Alliance Key #9 - Be Gentle with Yourself

Just in case I haven't yet gotten this message across, the single most important thing you can do to move beyond compulsive eating is to be gentle, understanding and compassionate with yourself. You now *know* that the harder you are on yourself, the more you will be drawn towards emotional eating to silence the critical and worried voice in your head. Alternately, having a loving inner dialogue is a not only a kind thing to do for yourself, but also a vital part of your weight-release process.

I know from reviewing my history with compulsive eating that the time I was most likely to come down hard on myself was immediately following a binge. I later learned that this was *also* the most important time to be deeply sympathetic with myself. When my inner dialogue became kinder, when I had a sweeter and more compassionate voice in my head, I was able to breathe through my urges to eat far more easily. It is *miraculous* what a difference this one self-loving practice can make.

It may take you a while to get into the groove of *Eating In Alliance* with your body. Every person has a different rate of progress. And when you keep your thoughts focused on the positive conviction that it will *absolutely* happen for you, it will. Perhaps not in the time frame that you had deemed ideal, but rather within the one that is appropriate for you given your specific relationship with food.

The practice of *Eating in Alliance* is just that, a *practice*—a process of repeating something many times. In order for your new eating behaviors to become permanent and second nature, you simply need to practice them over and over again. From the first time you breathe through the

217

urge to binge, you hold the "memory" of it in your body, a snapshot if you will. That's the picture or foundation from which your new relationship with your body will progress. The more times you repeat that "memory," of staying connected with your body as you eat, the easier *Eating in Alliance* becomes. You are re-training yourself to adopt a new and healthier behavior around food. I repeat: repetition is key! The more you practice and the more compassionate you are with your process, the faster you will reconnect with your body.

Keep in mind that your goal is not to *Eat in Alliance* one hundred percent of the time. That perfectionist goal virtually guarantees disappointment and frustration. Shooting for eighty to ninety percent is a much smarter goal. The change from compulsive to connected eating is not often like a light switch you can flip. Rather it is a series of conscious choices that you make, one after the other. If you practice the *Eating in Alliance Keys* even ten percent of the time during your first few weeks, it is HUGE! Expecting your habits to change overnight is harmful to your ability to see how far you have come. Give yourself credit for each and every tiny step you take towards your goal to reconnect with your body.

Learning to *Eat in Alliance* was a very gradual process for me. It felt like it snuck up on me. I was surprised and thrilled when I turned a corner in my relationship with food and I was able to wait, without even thinking about it, until I was legitimately hungry to eat. At the later stages of my recovery I remember thinking to myself, "Wow, I didn't think about eating compulsively almost all day today. I can't *believe* it! It's a miracle!" This was an extraordinarily liberating feeling for me, and you can feel it too. Your recovery process may be gradual, but it is a certainty. To support your intention to be gentle with yourself, think of progress and not perfection on your journey. If it happens overnight, fantastic! However, for most of us it takes a bit longer to create a new relationship with food.

The poet Robert Lewis Stevenson said, "Remember to judge each day not by the harvest you reap, but by the seeds you plant." I love this quote because it reminds me to acknowledge myself for anything I do, every little thing, because each action is a seed that eventually bears some form of a sweet fruit.

Alliance Key #10 - Make the Program Uniquely Yours

The final key, making the program uniquely yours, refers to the importance of defining for yourself what specific behaviors and boundaries allow you to experience the greatest level of success in your process of creating peace around food. There may be an additional guideline or key that you want to add to the above list to make it your own. Some women will find tremendous success by following the *Alliance Keys* and then adding an extra key that makes them feel more in control.

Here's an example. I know one woman who allows herself to eat anything she wants with the exception of candy and desserts because sugar sends her into an eating frenzy that is hard to escape. Sugar is a drug. (And as a side note, it's the only food that you can set on fire!) It is a highly addictive substance, so this woman allows herself natural sugars, but no processed sugars, so she doesn't feel totally confined. This additional tool has served her ability to eat in connection with her body extremely well. In part because she has given herself permission to eat anything else she wants, she feels empowered to make the choice to give up a food(s) that triggers her compulsions.

I personally don't have a single boundary around food. I eat anything I choose. I experimented with limiting my sugar intake, but restricting myself in that way made me feel confined and even more attracted to the forbidden sweets. However, you are a unique individual and must find out for yourself what serves you best in your journey to a healthier relationship with food. You alone can determine what boundaries will allow you to feel supported in your process. This may require some experimentation as you explore your response to eliminating particular foods, as you test yourself to determine what works for you. There is no "wrong" way if it feels right to your body. Although many compulsive overeaters need to allow themselves complete freedom to eat *whatever* they choose, others need a stronger boundary in order to feel free from their tendency to eat compulsively. Sometimes freedom comes through setting a boundary that makes you feel more in control, more empowered.

If there is a "trigger" food that you know *always* sends you into a state in which you are devouring food unconsciously, allow yourself to experiment with setting a boundary of *your* choosing when or if you will eat it. If the restriction makes you want it more, legalize it with all the other foods. Trust your guidance. Follow your heart. Tailor the program to your unique self, by choosing *for yourself* which supportive guidelines to follow.

The Comprehensive Plan

The way this program is structured is that each *Alliance* key builds on the others. By integrating even a *few* of the keys, you will turn your tide towards an increasingly connected relationship with your body. You don't have to use all of them at the same time to benefit from each one independently. For example, if you decide to eat when you are not hungry, rather than judging yourself for it, just be sure to use all the *other* keys. This will be a giant step in the right direction. It will allow you to really enjoy what you are eating, and you will be more likely to stop eating compulsively much sooner. If you eat beyond a Stage Six, you can still pat yourself on the back if you sat down while you ate, took three conscious breaths before eating, ate without distractions or drank a glass of water. Taking *any* of these actions will move you closer to connecting with your body and overcoming habitual eating.

Success Synopsis

Listed next is a summary of the reasons that diets don't work and why *Eating in Alliance* with your body does. Post it somewhere where you will see it regularly as a constant reminder as to why *Eating in Alliance* with your body is the smartest choice you can make!

221

Eating in Alliance	Dieting
*A Natural Approach	*An Artificial Approach
*Able to eat any food you want	*Limits food selections
*Reconnects you with your body	*Disconnects you from your body
*Creates healthy relationship with food	*Creates obsession with food
*Long-term approach	*Ineffective quick-fix approach
*Creates freedom around food	*Creates fear around food
*Effective weight loss technique	*Ineffective method
*Healthy for your body	*Unhealthy for your body
*Promotes trust of your body	*Creates distrust of your body
*Creates optimal health and energy	*Creates an artificial famine
*Guides you to eat when hungry	*Teaches you to ignore hunger
*Creates healthy relationship with food	*Creates dysfunction
*Honors your body	*Confuses your body
*Creates optimal energy	*Exhausts your body
*Reduces emotional eating	*Intensifies emotional eating
*Inspires you to trust yourself	*Keeps you in a state of distrust
*Fosters self-acceptance	*Induces judgment & frustration
*Results in weight loss	*Results in weight gain

*****

222

Exercise is to your health what shutting your eyes is to sleeping."

– Anonymous

Chapter 6

Exercise and You

The Natural High

I'm just going to say it straight and rip the band-aid off as quickly as possible. If you want to be the healthiest you can be, exercise *has* to become a consistent part of your life. There is no getting around it. Did you get a sinking feeling when you read that statement? Did you feel trapped? Does the thought of going to a gym make you break out in hives? Many of us cringe when we think of working out because we think it will be a boring or worse, a highly uncomfortable experience.

But before your untamed mind latches onto these thoughts in an effort to keep you couch-bound, I want to *assure* you that exercise can also be enjoyable, especially when you find a form that works for you and your body. This is not solely because of the rush of "feel good" chemicals (endorphins) that are released in your body when you exert yourself physically, but *also* because the positive mental boost that occurs when you *know* you have done something good for your body is, in and of itself, a very generous "high." And in response to exercise, your glorious, pleasure-oriented body rewards you for doing something healthy by making you feel better, much better, both physically and emotionally. It seems to be the body's way of saying, "Hey, thank you for taking care of me, I really appreciate it."

As we've already explored in depth, body love is an integral component of self-love given that your body houses your "self." And the very self-loving practice of exercise affirms, in a very tangible way, your intention to connect with and take care of your body. Just as you might feel loved if someone bought you flowers, your body feels loved when you use it, when you keep it active rather than letting it atrophy.

But the practice of exercise offers *much* more than just physical benefits. The *mental* benefits that accompany it are just as numerous. One benefit is that working out gets you *used* to feeling uncomfortable regularly as you push yourself physically. Learning to embrace temporary physical discomfort is an important goal for compulsive eaters who usually avoid discomfort like they would a ferocious dog. Exercise helps you to increase your tolerance for discomfort. It is a profound training in learning how to deal with uncomfortable feelings head-on. As you train yourself to endure discomfort physically through exercise, you heighten your ability to tolerate the emotional discomfort that often results in a binge. Remember, you've experienced a lot of discomfort already and you are still here to tell the story.

Exercise helps you to understand that discomfort, whether mental or physical, can be managed and mastered. It also is a powerful reminder that uncomfortable times are *always* temporary! Your feelings can change like the tides in a moment's time. Can you think of a time when you were upset about something, but then got distracted and your frustration dissipated? Maybe you were in a bad traffic jam feeling like you wanted to scream your head off one minute and then you heard your favorite song and instantly you were singing your little heart out. Instant mood change! Our untamed minds, like little children, can almost always be distracted by more appealing thoughts or activities. Exercise helps you to learn how to deal with your uncomfortable emotions, to resist the urge to binge like you would resist the urge to quit the workout. Fortunately, your surrender to the discomfort, whether emotional or physical, actually reduces its intensity. You deflate the feelings by sticking with them until they lessen and gradually evaporate.

After a period of pushing yourself beyond your comfort zone by sticking with your exercise program, you'll begin to experience a more empowered state of mind. In this positive state, you'll start to realize that you can accomplish anything you set your mind to. You'll start to be impressed with yourself, which generates a more positive incentive to continue your practice of exercise. Any step you take towards being more physically active is a great idea. Whether it's taking the stairs instead of the escalator, or vacuuming with gusto, acknowledge yourself for each physical activity. It will keep you motivated to push yourself a little further each time when you appreciate even the most modest of improvements!

Awareness Opportunity

Take a moment to look at the following list of life priorities, choose your top ten and then rank them in order of importance.

Success

Wealth

Love

Comfort

Family

Health

Power

Freedom

Education

Adventure

Fame

Passion

Creativity

Contribution

Fun

Safety

Honesty

Intelligence

Growth

Security

Intimacy

Education

Happiness

Peace

Where did health appear in your list of priorities?

Do you think you would be able to enjoy any of your other priorities, whether it is fame or passion or even tremendous wealth, if you were sick?

What form of exercise are you most attracted to today on any level?

It is important to take the time to prioritize your values – specifically so that you can experience your most important ones daily. I didn't define my priorities and rank them in order of importance until my early thirties, which is why it took me so darn long to get my life to reflect what I most wanted! When I clearly defined my health as one of my top priorities, it inspired me to take action to honor this value more consistently, taking it to the forefront of my attention where I could no longer deny its significance. Exercise is now a non-negotiable activity I engage in as much as possible, and I love doing it (most of the time).

Finding the time to exercise can seem challenging at first, but when it becomes a top priority, you will get highly creative insights into how to make it happen. You'll bargain with your husband, beg your mother and trade off with friends to fit it in. There's always a way to make it happen, even if you work full time and are raising a family. If you have children, you can walk them in a jogger or you can dance with them in the family room or in your backyard in the fresh air. You can workout in the privacy of your home with DVDs or take walks around your neighborhood. Being committed to exercise will be a healthy example if you have children who will benefit from establishing early patterns of being physically active. If you work a full-time job, you can take a walk with a co-worker during lunch or immediately after work. Weekends will provide you with an opportunity for some physical activity if your weeks are chock-full. Should you have a significant other, ask for their support. Explain to them that *both* of you will benefit when you are taking better care of your body because you'll be an even happier person.

Even if you increase your heart rate for half an hour a day three to five times a week, it can and will make all the difference in the world to your physical and mental well-being. You will get addicted to the wonderful feeling that exercise generates relatively quickly. Your body was designed to be active, which is why we feel so great after we have gotten into a regular physical practice. Even a little exercise can have a positive impact on your health!

Here's another benefit of exercise: it is a powerful antidote to melancholy. If you find yourself down and depressed and you want to feel better, get physical! Move that body in any way that you can. And when exercise is coupled with spending time outdoors in Mother Nature, you get a double bang for your buck because exercising outdoors is a powerful antidote for mild depression as well. In a study at Britain's Essex University, researchers had people who were suffering from depression take a thirty-minute walk. Some walked in a wooded park and others in an indoor shopping center. After the country walk, seventy-one percent said they felt less depressed, and ninety percent said it made them feel better about themselves. After the shopping-center walk, on the other hand, only forty-five percent felt less depressed, and twenty-two percent said they felt more depressed. Another forty-four percent said their self-esteem had fallen (I remember that day-in-the-mall shopping slump all too well). Spending too much time indoors will depress you. It is simply not natural if you are not balancing it with time outdoors.

Think about it in these terms, although our culture now predominantly lives indoors (we work, sleep, eat, drive and frequently exercise indoors), it has not always been the way. Most jobs used to be agriculturally oriented and entire days were spent outside. There seems to be a correlation between the amount of time we spend indoors as a society and depression rates. So double your pleasure, both physical and mental. Whenever possible, spend time outside getting active, preferably someplace you find beautiful. It holds the power to change your life.

If you are exercising regularly you are going to increase your self-esteem, extend your lifespan, slow your aging process, increase your muscle tone and more easily release excess weight. And you can do it all for free! No creams, pills or operations necessary, thank you! What a bargain!

The Spotlight Effect

I know that many people don't exercise in part because they feel self-conscious. They are afraid that others are watching them and judging them for the shape or size of their bodies. They allow their fear that someone they do not know might have a judgmental thought about their bodies to stop them from doing something that is incredibly important to their health. I know this because I did the very same thing for years. The funny thing is that I would judge myself all day, every day and never even stop to notice, but if someone *else* did it to me, or even if I *thought* they were, I felt like I wanted the earth to swallow me up. I gave my power away to complete strangers, skipping exercise that I knew was good for me on the off chance that someone might stare at me or think ill of me. My innocent but false belief that people would spend their time fixating on my body kept me from taking better care of it by getting physical.

A Cornell University study explored this phenomenon of deep self-consciousness, which, not so surprisingly, is known as the "spotlight effect." It is the delusion that the world is paying close attention to us, far greater attention than is actually the case. In truth, say Cornell University researchers, you are generally ignored by others, and if noticed, not judged as harshly as you imagine. Take note and take heart!

Most often people are too dang busy judging themselves to spend their time judging you! It's more likely that you, like me, are projecting your constant judgment of yourself onto other people. If you are a victim of the "spotlight effect," you are most likely spending way too much energy suffering for no reason at all. Make *you* your priority rather than what others are (or are not) thinking about you.

It's important to remind yourself that your fear of being judged by others is activated by your trouble-making untamed mind. However, your untamed mind can be quickly muzzled when you repeatedly exercise and have a positive feeling affiliated with each experience. When you catch your untamed mind suggesting ridiculous things ("They're all going to stare at you!"), guide your inner dialogue in a smarter and kinder direction ("Honey, don't you worry about what anyone else thinks! You get your sweet body moving and don't give your power away by investing in what other people think.") On the remote chance that someone stops thinking about their own life long enough to judge you, your growth opportunity is to recognize that their judgments are being generated by their own untamed mind. If someone feels the need to judge you, it indicates that they simply feel inadequate about themselves on some level. Ignore their judgments and spend your energy investing in your well-being.

Getting Started

Start with a form of exercise that appeals to you above all others rather than the one you think will burn the most calories. Your exercise program *must* have some appealing aspects to it so that you look forward to it. So go for the fun right away. If you choose one or two forms of exercise that you enjoy on any level, you will be more likely to stick with them.

Being the "variety is the spice of life" type of a gal that I am, I choose a combination of exercises so that I keep my enthusiasm high. I do a few that get my heart rate up (tennis, fast walking, biking), and some that stretch and tone my body (yoga and weight lifting). My exercise regime is another opportunity for me to "put the world on hold" and take quality time out to connect with and care for my body and myself. I also find that after an intense workout, I am far choosier about what I eat. I remember thinking when I first started working out, "I didn't work *that* hard in my aerobics class just to blow it on this donut. No thanks! It's not worth it!"

I highly recommend working out with a partner or participating in a group exercise program when you are first starting so you can get into the groove with the support of others. Group exercise was a valuable resource for me because it was often highly motivating to see everyone around me, at all weights and shapes, moving their bodies. It intensified my commitment significantly. It is almost as though I caught the wave of strength flowing among all of my co-exercisers, which helped me to keep my energy up. If you are able to motivate yourself independent of anyone else's urgings and if you prefer to exercise alone, you still have plenty of wonderful options to reconnect you with your body.

Some forms of exercise are especially effective for reconnecting with your body. For me, yoga is one of them. I practice yoga two to three times a week, and it has been *pivotal* to my reconnection with my body. The translation of yoga is "union" and if you are looking to create a stronger union with your body, yoga is for you. Yoga is a form of exercise that strikes a rare balance between "being" and "doing." You alternate between moving through the yoga postures (doing) and staying as still as possible as you hold the yoga postures and focus on creating a peaceful state of mind (being). Studies show that yoga relieves stress, slows the aging process (a big draw for me), improves health (another substantial benefit), firms and tones (thank you) and builds strength. And the icing on the cake is that it can also support you in your weight-release goals! Yoga helps me to take a mental vacation from the responsibilities of my day so I can refocus my attention in the present moment, which always increases my feelings of well-being. Yoga also lowers the levels of the stress hormone cortisol, helps with blood pressure, heart rate, fatigue and insomnia. It offers a veritable smorgasbord of benefits!

Yoga has also supported me in improving my posture, which is important for a variety of reasons. If you chronically hunch your shoulders, slumping forward as you sit and stand, you are unintentionally constricting your heart, digestive organs and lungs. Yoga postures are designed to optimize your breathing, increasing oxygen to your bloodstream and boosting your overall energy. When you take deep breaths, you are sending a signal to your nervous system that it is time to relax. Yoga will help you to practice ideal posture and help you carry it into your life outside of your yoga sanctuary.

Something else that inspires me about yoga is that it is an incredible way to ensure that, in your golden years, you will have a level of flexibility, balance and strength. You are far less likely to sustain injury or have a chronically painful condition if you are flexible and agile. I don't know about you, but I want to slide into those golden years with every advantage available to me!

For the compulsive eater, one of the greatest benefits of yoga is that it provides a very strong and deliberate practice for breathing with, and through, discomfort. More so than any other physical activity I have tried, yoga helps me surrender to my feelings and breathe through my urges to binge. Staying with some of the challenging yoga postures allows you to "make peace with discomfort." In yoga practice, you assume specific poses and postures, some of which are challenging because they require both balance and strength. You use your breath and focused attention to help you relax your untamed mind, which is saying, "I can't hold it anymore," or "This is really uncomfortable," as you remain in the postures. You learn to quiet your untamed mind, to hold the poses for increasingly long periods of time as you build strength of body and strength of will. While you are in the process of moving into a yoga posture, you are gently directed by your teacher to breathe in synchronicity with each move. You get a "breath training" workshop in your yoga practice.

Again, the conscious breathing you will get trained on in yoga expands your ability to feel comfortable feeling uncomfortable. You learn to sooth your physical discomfort, and quiet your untamed mind, with your breath. Breathing optimally is a *massively* powerful technique for dissolving discomfort, whether it is the physical discomfort of the yoga posture or the emotional discomfort of challenging feelings. This form of exercise allows you to become more confident in your ability to "be" with discomfort and to reduce it through breathing in concert with high-vibration thinking. Skilled yoga instructors are as committed to training your breath as they are to training your body!

Yoga allowed me to expand my capacity to engage my willpower, to build my inner strength and my ability to breathe through intense, untamed mind-driven urges for food.

Your experience of yoga will be highly dependent upon the yoga instructor, which is why it is important to ask around for the one in your community who has a strong and positive reputation. And be sure to try out a few yoga classes to see which type most appeals to you. There are a variety of them including Ashtanga (an aerobic version of yoga), Iyengar (which involves holding postures for longer time frames) and Hatha (which focuses on stretching) to name a few.

Before I complete this pitch for yoga I would like to highlight a final benefit, one that, as an admitted pleasure junky, I adore. Yoga feels good – really, really good. Many of the twists and stretching exercises feel like you are giving yourself a wonderful internal and external massage. And after yoga practice you will experience a fully relaxed body and one of the most delicious natural highs you can imagine. Your body is being oxygenated, cleansed and energized as you participate in the practice and will give you yet another opportunity to see how much pleasure your body can provide when you partner with it.

The Wide Wide World of Sports

Okay, now I'm done with my yoga pitch. Let's get back to the wider range of exercise available to you! If you want your life to hold more excitement, be adventuresome in your choices! Try something new! Stretch yourself for the love of you! Whether it's Rollerblading or jumping rope, or walking around the block, start some form of physical activity that you are excited about this very day and it will likely become a healthy habit very quickly. The first few weeks are usually the toughest because you are going against the flow of the old way and transitioning to the new. But after the momentum of exercising regularly takes over, it's much, much easier. You have to push yourself past the hump.

When your untamed mind tries to make excuses for not exercising, remember that you have the power to coach yourself lovingly but firmly through that self-defeating voice. Take action, even if it is as modest as a twenty-minute walk around your neighborhood or a "private dance party" in your home to your favorite upbeat music. I can promise you, without reservation, that once you find your favorite form of exercise, you won't feel complete without it! If you knew you could win cash and prizes for exercising, would you be more motivated to do it? I know I would! And exercise will help you to win the ultimate prize, a healthier and more connected relationship with your body. Now *that's* priceless!

*****

"Together we can do so much." – Helen Keller

Chapter 7

Co-Coaching:

The Partnership Approach to Achieving Your Natural and Ideal Weight

The Birth of Co-Coaching

When I was living full-time with an eating disorder, one of the most painful aspects of my life was the extreme and constant sense of isolation I felt. Even though I was very active socially, I felt totally alone in my addiction. I could be at a great party, surrounded by people I was crazy about and whom I knew loved me and yet *still* feel disconnected from the celebration because of the critical dialogue going on in my untamed mind. *"Don't eat that. I wonder if he would like me if I wasn't overweight? What are they thinking about the fact that I have packed on the pounds? God help me, I want to eat that entire apple cobbler, and throw in that caramel chunk cheese cake while I'm at it."*

I had family and friends who genuinely wanted to support me in my struggle to release weight, but my internalized shame prevented me from reaching out for help. I only told those closest to me that I was unhappy with my body, and *no* one knew I was bulimic. I was far too embarrassed to share those intimate details with anyone. But in the deepest part of my being, I longed for a partner, someone who could comfort me as I breathed through my urges to overeat, who would inspire me to be strong when I felt weak and help me get over my compulsion with food once and for all. "Please, please, please," I begged the Divine. "Help me get beyond this. I just don't think I can do it alone."

In spite of the humiliation I felt about my inability to control what I ate, my increasing desperation *finally* led me to break down and approach my close girlfriend, Helen, for support. Remember Helen from Chapter 6, my childhood friend who lived across the street? Well, twenty years later I was living directly below her in the same apartment building. One day when we were hanging out talking, I couldn't hold it in anymore and I shared with her the depths of my unhappiness with my body and a little bit about my compulsion with food. Even though Helen had never faced a weight challenge or food obsession, she was enormously compassionate (she is one of the sweetest people I have ever met). It felt *really* good to open up even a little bit to a friend. I felt some of my burden lift simply because Helen was so kind, empathetic and nonjudgmental. She made me feel so comfortable that I went out on a limb and decided to ask for her support. Specifically, I asked her to help me stay on a diet that I had heard was guaranteed to make me lose at least ten pounds in ten days.

Because she didn't know that diets don't work either, Helen readily agreed to be my personal coach and was genuinely enthusiastic about helping me. I was really excited about getting started because I thought that the combination of her support and the newest "miracle quick weight loss program" would be the answer to my most fervent and desperate prayers.

The day before we began the program, I bought all the food the diet called for plus some of my favorite foods at that time: yogurt-covered raisins, Little Debbie's glazed donuts and cheese pizza. When I got home, I hastily put away all the diet foods and then gorged myself on the foods I considered bad. If I was going to have to eat diet food for the next ten days, I was going to have a "last supper," by golly. Predictably, I went to bed miserably full, stuffed to capacity, a sickening Stage Ten.

The next day I walked up to Helen's apartment and knocked on her door. Although I felt a little nauseated from the prior night's binge, hope still sprang eternal for me as I thought about the new diet. That is, until I handed Helen the written version of the diet to check out. I can distinctly remember the startled look on her face as she read off the first day's breakfast menu, "Two pieces of dried toast and a half a grapefruit." Having never been on a diet herself, she looked at me with an expression of complete disbelief. "This is all you *get*?" she exclaimed. "That's *crazy*, it's no wonder you can't stay on a diet!"

Thinking she might back out of our arrangement, I begged her to stick with me, making all sorts of excuses for the meager portions and bland food options because I was desperate for her assistance. Although she was highly dubious as to the wisdom of my diet, she reluctantly agreed to continue helping me. Every morning Helen gave me a pep talk, reminding me of how good it was going to feel to reach my goal weight. I'd call her while I was at work and I'd share with her my urges to abandon the diet and she'd inspire me to keep my eye on the ball (she was a nationally ranked tennis player). Knowing that she was invested in my success made it easier for me to stick to the diet. I felt like I was a part of a team rather than a lone wolf.

At night we would marvel and laugh over the bland menus I was allowed, and she would urge me to be strong and think "long-term" satisfaction. She reminded me that the diet was only ten days of "palate torture" in exchange for reaching my weight-release goal. Helen made the process easier and more enjoyable than any other diet I had ever been on, and I did in fact lose nine pounds in ten days. But, predictably, I gained it all back, plus an additional five pounds, once I returned to my normal eating habits. It took me another six years to figure out that it was the diet, not my willpower, that was the problem. Regardless of Helen's incredible support, and because neither one of us knew the dangers and ineffectiveness of dieting, I had been doomed from the start. Nonetheless, through this experience, I learned the incredible power of partnership and the co-coaching seed was planted (more on that to come).

In 1994, I entered into my second coaching relationship with a woman named Jackie Priestley. Jackie had worked through her own compulsive eating disorder and had started a coaching practice to guide men and women to reconnect with their true physical appetites and reach their goal weight the natural way, by listening to their bodies. At our first session, I felt an immediate connection and I was sure I wanted to work with her. I felt relieved to have *finally* met a person who could relate intimately to every aspect of my battle with food, diets and disconnection from my body. I could speak to Jackie without feeling self-conscious because she understood *everything* I had gone through: the out-of-control binges, the body shame and the intense frustration of trying to release weight. She appreciated how very challenging the process of healing a food addiction could be and provided an incredibly effective environment for my healing to begin taking place. She was fun, kind, compassionate and offered *fantastic* support and guidance.

Supported by Jackie's coaching, I progressed in my awareness of my own relationship with my body and, indeed, myself. We met once a week for about a year, though given the severity of my compulsive relationship with food, I really needed to meet with her every day. I left each coaching session excited about what I had learned about myself and eager to try the tools she gave me. Yet when I left her office, I was frequently drawn back into my compulsive eating patterns almost immediately. I knew in my heart that the non-dieting approach to releasing weight was the way to go, yet actually *doing* it was still highly challenging. I felt that if I could have talked to her in those moments when I was faced with the urge to eat, she would have been able to talk me out of it. She could have inspired me to breathe through the urge to binge. That was not an option for me at that time.

What I desperately wanted, what I desperately needed, was to feel comfortable enough with someone to call them up in those shaky moments when I could feel myself gravitating towards the kitchen and say, "Hey, I'm tempted to binge right now and I'm not even hungry. Do you have a minute? Could you please talk me out of it?" I couldn't imagine saying anything like that to even my closest friends. I would have been far too embarrassed.

Ultimately it was admitting the severity of my problem to Jackie during our sessions that proved to be the first step in moving beyond it. I had to get brave, to share my deepest, darkest secrets around my compulsive eating disorder. I found immense internal freedom in my full disclosure to someone who was invested in my getting over my obsession with eating.

What I now know is that any one of us would have a *far* greater chance of healing our compulsion with food if we had a full-time coach, especially in the early stages of recovery. In this modern day world where addiction of one sort or another is pretty much the norm, we *all* need support in one way or another. To pretend we don't is self-defeating. So if you are having a hard time and want to progress quickly in healing your compulsion, it is a smart idea to stop choosing door number one (flying solo) when door number two (partnering up) gives you access to the friendly skies of freedom around food.

Would you like to have support right in the moment (or darn close to it) when you are tempted to eat? Can you imagine having a voice of reason to counterbalance the "Me want more food" voice in your own head?

The concept and practice of co-coaching was created for this very reason.

Introducing Co-Coaching

Co-coaching is a partnership in which you and a chosen friend guide, support, motivate, challenge and inspire one other to achieve a specific goal. (In this chapter I am writing under the assumption that the co-coaching relationship will be between two women. This will not always be the case. It can just as easily take place between a man and a woman, or even two men. I'm writing from the single perspective for simplification purposes only).

In this case, your goal is to develop a healthy relationship with food and to learn to *Eat in Alliance* with your body. If you choose to go the partnership route, you will team up with another person (a friend, co-worker, family member) who is also struggling with emotional appetites and weight in order to support each other to move beyond addictive eating patterns. In a co-coaching relationship, you and your partner will make yourselves available to each other regularly to assist each other in transcending the urge to overeat. You will be sounding boards and guidance counselors, offering helpful suggestions to each other for alternative ways to calm and nurture yourself. You will also be reminding one another of all the ways that you will each benefit from waiting to eat until you are hungry. Your co-coach will also be personally invested in your goals and committed to supporting you in achieving them, and you will do the same for your co-coach.

As co-coaches, you will encourage each other when you are feeling down and frustrated. You will help each other learn to ignore the untamed mind when it says, "I want another heaping serving." You will guide each other to access a loving internal dialogue that will help you overcome binge eating. You will share suggestions and resources, commiserate with each other's struggles, encourage each other to make the healthiest choices available and give each other a much-needed nudge or hug when necessary.

Your co-coach will root you on when you feel stuck, remind you of your goals, inspire you to stick with the practice and listen to you empathetically when you are feeling overwhelmed. She will help you discover, understand, accept and love who you are today, identify and clarify what you want most in your future, and develop strategies to achieve your goals. She will help guide you to a deeper understanding of what, specifically, is driving your binge urges, support you in diffusing the energy around the urges and encourage you to choose a healthy alternative to eating to nurture yourself. Don't you love her already! And she'll feel the same because you will do the same for her!

Please note, however, that as beneficial as the co-coaching relationship can be, your co-coach *cannot* take the place of a professional counselor or medical doctor. If you have an intensely compulsive relationship with food, are bulimic or anorexic, or are using diuretics, laxatives or amphetamines to control your weight, you need to be under the care of a professional. It is a mandatory component in your healing. It would be unfair and unhealthy to expect your partner to assume the role of therapist or doctor. Having the support of your co-coach *and* a therapist and/or doctor, on the other hand, would be a highly beneficial combination.

It is obvious that you will benefit from having a coach. I mean, what isn't easier and more fun when it is done with a beloved friend?! You are looking to master eating in connection with your body, and virtually *all* masters—whether they be concert pianists, professional athletes, master painters or famous opera singers—get support and lots of it! Having a coach is simply the wisest thing you can do to expedite your progress.

But what about being a coach to someone else? You might be thinking, "Gee, Lily, that's great. I'm all for helping others, but I'm just trying to learn how to help myself right now. How can I help someone else? Why should I?" Here's the answer. To teach is to learn and to learn is to teach.

As you coach your partner, you will, at the same time, help yourself and naturally accelerate your own ability to *Eat in Alliance* with your body. It is the *ultimate* win-win. When you coach your partner to breathe through the urge to eat, you hone your own ability to guide yourself through the same urges. When your friend is breathing through an urge to binge, you will bring your most loving, firm and encouraging voice to assist her. You will remind her of the many ways she will benefit from overcoming the urge to binge; you will remind her of the price she pays for listening to her untamed mind; you will remind her, "Yes, you can do it!" With time and practice, you will learn to turn that same gentle and encouraging voice on yourself. The more you offer her this coaching gift, the more it will become engrained in both of your personal psyches. The more you coach your partner, the more you will understand how to move through compulsive eating desires on your own. When she is not available to you because of other commitments, you will remember what you told *her* and simply offer yourself the same sage guidance!

Part of the extra incentive you will feel as a co-coach comes from the awareness that the process of recovery is about more than just *you*. It is also about your partner, which interestingly offers you a sense of relief. You are now a team, and part of what happens when you commit to the partnership is that you are more likely to think long and hard before you break a commitment to yourself. Whereas in the past you might have caved in to the urge to eat compulsively right away, you'll now have a reason to hesitate, to stop and center yourself. That reason is your partner. It is simply easier to stay committed to a common goal when more than just your own interests are at stake.

Just as making a commitment to another person *substantially* increases your individual chances of success, helping others enhances your self-image. When you do kind, loving things, it is easier to love yourself, and the more you love yourself, the more your emotional appetites diminish. The feeling of internal fullness you feel makes breathing through compulsive eating much, much easier.

So just for fun, let me summarize the benefits of having and being a co-coach:

-When you partner with another individual, you dramatically improve your ability to reconnect with your body to achieve your natural weight.

-Partnership makes your process more interesting and fun, and whenever lightness and joy are involved in any activity, it naturally becomes easier.

-Partnership takes the isolating effects out of your process.

-Partnership provides a built-in support structure to move you through the difficult times.-

-Partnership offers additional incentive to break through compulsive eating urges for the benefit of the "team."

-As you share feedback with each other and guide each other along the way, you will gain significant insights into yourself and your partner. This opens the door for greater levels of intimacy.

-Partnership helps you to learn how to be your own coach and greatest ally.

-Partnership builds your sense of self and self-esteem by helping someone else.

The Co-Coaching Relationship

The first thing you want to do to start your co-coaching relationship is to choose a partner. Do you know someone who is struggling with her/his own body or food issues? Do you have a close friend, relative or partner that you would feel comfortable approaching for support? Keep in mind that your co-coach does not have to have eating issues to support you – they simply have to be invested in your success. In most cases, the person you will choose to partner with is already a friend and a source of comfort, joy and fun in your life. This new co-coaching relationship will be a natural extension of the support you already offer each other in your friendship. In some cases, you may have to look outside of your circle of friends to find the right fit. Be open-minded in your search. I guarantee that there is an ideal partner out there who will be *incredibly* grateful to team up with you!

Once you have agreed to partner with this individual, the next step is to define the duration of your co-coaching relationship. I highly recommend making a commitment to each other for a minimum of one month because research has shown that it requires about that length of time to integrate a new habit. Why not give yourself every possible advantage?

This next step is to define your "check-in" schedule, a time(s) during the day when you will connect with each other to keep each other focused, inspired and excited. While the most important time to be available for each other is during the urge to binge, there are other times to check in that will support you in staying motivated and focused.

At the beginning of your co-coaching relationship, I suggest checking in first thing in the morning and once in the evening at mutually agreed-upon times. Before your morning phone call, spend five quiet minutes in meditation and then, from this centered space, create a personal intention for yourself for your day. This intention may be to say only loving things to yourself all day. It may be that you are committed to watching your thoughts, or that you will do your very best to follow through on all the *Eating in Alliance* keys. When you connect with your co-coach for your morning call, communicate your personal intention to her along with anything else that feels like it wants to be shared.

At this time you can get one another pumped up with a "You can do it!" inspirational conversation. If you both have time, you can download your untamed mind's worries to each other and help one another find a high-vibration perspective or solution to challenges you are each facing. These coaching conversations will serve to diminish your emotional appetites, which will, in turn, make navigating your day that much easier. During your evening check-in call, share with your partner what worked for you during that day to help you stay connected to your body and the personal successes you experienced as well as the tools you used to support yourself in transcending the urge to binge.

During the thirty days, in addition to the mutually agreed-upon check in conversations in the morning and evening, there will be "support" calls. Any time either you or your partner are tempted to eat when not physically hungry, you can pick up the phone and call each other for support and inspiration. Before calling however, please use at least one of the self-empowerment techniques in Chapter 8 on your own. It is important that you call your partner when you absolutely know for *sure* that you cannot breathe through the urge to binge by yourself. You don't want to create a relationship in which you are so dependent on your partner that you don't put in an effort to help yourself first. In the very beginning it is likely that there will be quite a few support calls made back and forth, and that is common and totally appropriate. You are learning the new skill of *Eating in Alliance* and that requires time, practice and patience. Just stretch yourself a little bit more each time, putting in a few minutes of deep-relaxation breathing and high-vibration thinking prior to picking up the phone. You'll be building your willpower muscle every time you do so!

During a support call, you can use your own model for lovingly assisting one another in breathing through the urge; you can also refer to the co-coaching dialogue model below that is guaranteed to support your partner in gaining clarity around her situation and choosing her best option given her circumstances.

The actual co-coaching dialogue that you will engage in is a simple one that consists of questions and gentle invitations. These coaching questions are designed to support your partner in determining what disempowering "story" her untamed mind is telling her. The invitations will allow her to access a loving, compassionate nurturing inner dialogue and come back to the present moment, where she will experience greater levels of peace and clarity. From this place she can decide whether or not she is going to choose to eat.

Coaching Dialogue Process:

1. What are you feeling (e.g., anger, sadness, fear, anxiety, guilt) right now?

2. Where is the feeling showing up in your body? (Invite her to place her hand on that spot and take three deep and expansive breaths right into the feeling. After a minute or so when she is feeling a little more centered

and relaxed, move on to the next question.)

3. What was the thought (situation) that created that feeling? (Listen attentively to her perspective then invite her to access her "sweet" internal voice as she answers the following question.)

4. What is the most powerful, loving and positive thought you can have right now to override the disempowering thought(s) that is causing you to feel this way? (Examples: There is no situation that I cannot handle. I have the ability to create anything I want in my life. I will love myself through this process, and know that I don't have to be perfect.) Or, What would be the most loving, high-vibration perspective you can have on your circumstances? (Listen to her attentively, then move on to the next question.)

5. What do you stand to gain if you choose an alternative to eating? (Listen attentively, then ask the following question.)

6. Which tool are you going to use to support yourself in staying centered and calm? (See Chapter 8 – Nurturing Alternatives to Eating). Or, How can I best support you in this moment? And finally, ask…

7. Do you feel you can you wait to eat until you are hungry? If the answer is "no," simply remind her to use all the other *Eating Alliance Keys*.

You can see that, as the coach, your predominant role will be to *ask* the questions and listen attentively to your partner. I know from experience that having someone to talk to in the middle of an urge is *incredibly* helpful. Just having Jackie or Helen listen and empathize with my concerns relaxed me and lessened the emotional appetites that were leading me towards a binge. Having someone listen to your concerns will often be more than enough to silence your untamed mind and create an internal sense of peace as you transcend the urge to eat when you are not hungry. Your attention to your feelings combined with your partner's attention to *you* is where the transformation takes place. Just being with your feelings as an alternative to reaching for food is a prime opportunity to befriend your feelings so that you no longer feel intimidated by them. With your partner's help, rather than resisting your feelings, you will gradually embrace them and allow them to communicate where an imbalance of thinking (untamed mind) or behavior (e.g., overworking, compulsive eating, overspending) is keeping you from being at peace with yourself and life. Rather than escaping your body, you learn to inhabit it along with its full spectrum of feelings, which are the ways your body suggests that you would benefit from making some shifts.

There will, of course, be times when your partner is not available to take a support call because of work, family obligations or other personal commitments and during those times Chapter 9 (The Self-Empowerment Chapter—Nurturing Alternatives to Eating) is your best resource.

As a side note, I highly recommend in advance defining times when it will *not* work for you to take a support call from your partner. Having clear boundaries around this aspect of co-coaching will help you to avoid confusion and frustration in your relationship. If mornings are bad for you because you are getting your children off to school, make it clear. It is a self-loving behavior for each of you to honor your boundaries, and having both parties define their ideal check-in schedule in advance is a smart start.

Confidentiality is, of course, a given in your co-coaching relationship. And, remember that your role is not only to be honest with your partner, but *gentle* and understanding in your feedback and interactions. This will create a safe space where she feels comfortable sharing her most intimate thoughts with you without fear of your judgment or frustration. Tremendous healing takes place in this domain.

Oh, and of course have *fun* creating your co-coaching partnership. Have a set kickoff date where you define your goals and commitments for the next thirty days and start your co-coaching relationship off with a meaningful ritual that establishes your purpose to reconnect with your body powerfully. On your inaugural date, have each coach sign the following coaching commitment as a final testament to your self-loving intentions!

Co-Coaching Commitment

I, (Your Name Here)commit to being a supportive Co-Coach to my partner.

Date:

In my role as co-coach:

1. I will create a non-judgmental and supportive environment for my partner.

2. I will offer advice only when asked or given permission.

3. I will consistently listen to my co-coach with an open heart.

4. I will offer my unconditional support.

5. I will honor the confidentiality of all information we share.

6. I will communicate my feelings and observations openly and honestly.

7. I will make the process a fun and enjoyable experience.

8. I will support _____ in seeing her own magnificence at any weight.

9. I will only talk in positive terms about my own body and the bodies of others.

10. I will honor all commitments I make to my co-coach or renegotiate them promptly.

11. I will allow my partner the space to experience her own process.

12. I will respect and honor my partner's needs that have been communicated.

13. I will support my partner in only speaking in positive terms about herself and will honor myself in the same way.

14. I commit to following the *Eating in Alliance* keys to the best of my ability and support my partner in doing the same.

*****

The caged bird longs to leave,

and the door is open

but it doesn't know it can fly out.

-Swami Yogananda

Chapter 8

Self-Empowerment Tools

Nurturing Alternatives to Eating

As you are first practicing *Eating in Alliance*, there will be times when a non-hunger related urge to eat tries to sink its teeth into you like a tick on a dog. When that happens, where are you to turn? To the self-empowerment chapter! This chapter is filled with techniques that you can turn to in an emergency, when you need assistance in transcending an urge to binge. Familiarize yourself with each of them and then try them out to see which one or which few work best for you.

Empowerment Options:

There are three main ways (options) to handle an urge to binge. You can:

1. Allow yourself to feel the feelings that are stimulating the urge to eat,

and open your heart to understand what is driving the urge to eat (e.g., need for down time, tenderness, fun, a release from stress, a prompting to take action). Your understanding of what is driving the binge should support you to create a calmer state of mind, which will assist you in waiting for the urge to pass, like a wave on the ocean. Keep in mind that every emotion has a purpose, a message and a limited life span.

2.   Allow yourself to eat, and follow the remainder of the *Eating in Alliance* keys to the best of your ability, giving your undivided attention to your food.

3.   Take action to overcome the urge by using one of the tools in this chapter.

The ideal choice is to surrender to your feelings, sitting and breathing through your uncomfortable feelings in order to determine what they are attempting to tell you. My own attempts to avoid or hold my feelings at bay by overeating ended up creating the very thing I was trying to avoid, more uncomfortable feelings that came with over-stuffing my body. I ended up creating circumstances in which I had no *choice* but to feel. Your soul *knows* that feelings, especially the hard ones, drive you inward. That internal journey is where we evolve and mature, it is the place where we break free of a limiting cocoon, spread our wings and take flight into a life that is bigger, more interesting and richer than we had ever imagined.

So, given this truth, ideally you will become intimate with your feelings and choose Option One. However, this sometimes just feels *too* intense. On those occasions, you need some alternatives. Listed below are tools

I use to get to an empowered state where I am able to say no to food that I am really not hungry for in the first place.

Empowering Toolbox

Depending upon your schedule, marital and job status, you will have varying time frames within which to overcome a binge. Sometimes you will need a tool that can help you when you are in a big pinch for time. At other times, you will have more time and space to get to the core of what is driving your urge to eat. Some of the tools will bring you to a state of harmony in your body and calm your untamed mind. From this state of peace you will be able to make healthy conscious choices about whether or not you want to eat. Other tools will provide you with a healthy and fun distraction that you can enjoy until the urge passes. Still others are just meant to put a little time and space between you and the food.

Try to find one or two tools that work best for you and stick with them. It can be more effective than bouncing from tool to tool because your familiarity with individual tools will allow you to default to it naturally with time. You'll build automatic and effective empowerment techniques when you are struck by a non-hunger related urge to eat.

Tool #1: Breathing Exercise

Relaxation breathing is one of the best things you can do to quiet the clamor in your untamed mind and thereby reduce the anxiety that promotes compulsive overeating. Poet Elizabeth Barrett Browning's quote: "He who breathes deepest lives longest," underscores beautifully the healthy effects of deep breathing. Deep breathing will slow you down and relax you, allowing you to engage your will to breathe through the urge to binge. It suspends your untamed mind's endless stream of negative thought so you can focus on all of the ways that you will benefit from allowing yourself to live at your natural weight. Here's what to do:

Sit in a chair with your back straight and your feet planted on the floor, ideally in a quiet and private space. Gently close your eyes and put your hands over your stomach with the tips of your fingers facing in towards your belly button. As you breathe in – as slowly as possible – through your nose, allow your breath to fill your stomach. You should feel a noticeable expansion throughout your rib cage and stomach. Direct your breath to fill your stomach first rather than puffing out your chest. The breaths that fill your abdomen are the ones that have the greatest relaxation impact. Your belly should feel like a beach ball being slowly inflated under your hands. There should be minimal movement in your upper chest area. Exhale through your nose, slowly and completely until you have no breath left. Repeat this cleansing breath three times.

Next, allow yourself to practice the following breathing pattern. Breathe in through your nose for four counts, hold your breath for four counts and then release your breath slowly and gently to the count of eight. Repeat this exercise eight times (or more if you wish) until you and your body feel more relaxed. Check in to see how you feel following the process. Do you feel calmer? More centered? More at peace? Breathing in a rhythmic pattern such as this one can support you in creating a sense of internal calm that will allow you to make a conscious adult choice about eating rather than making a childlike and impulsive decision from a state of emotional upset.

Tool # 2: Craving-Control Exercise

The next breathing technique we are going to practice is an alternative nostril breathing. Alternative nostril breathing calms your untamed mind, relaxes your body, increases your energy levels, improves your overall mood and even gives you a natural high. It is a breathing technique that has proven to be exceptionally powerful for conquering addictions and it has been around for a long, long time.

This technique is most effective if you are comfortably seated in an upright position with your eyes closed or downcast. Begin by placing the thumb of your dominant hand on one side of your nose and your index finger on the other side. Close off the nostril next to your index finger by pressing on it gently, just enough to close off the airflow.

Begin with a slow out-breath through the nostril closest to your thumb, feeling the air empty from your lungs as you exhale completely. Now take a deep and slow in-breath through that same nostril. Next, close off that nostril gently with your thumb, lift your index finger off your alternate nostril and exhale slowly and gently through that nostril. When you reach the point where you can't exhale any more air, take a deep in breath through that same nostril. Next, gently close off that nostril with your index finger and lift your thumb off your other nostril. Release your breath through the nostril closest to your thumb slowly and evenly and take an equally slow and even breath in through that nostril. With a little practice this breathing technique will be quite simple. Simply stated it is a back and forth inhale and exhale from nostril to nostril.

Continue this breathing pattern as long as necessary to calm your body and move past the non-hunger related eating urge. With each inhale, focus on becoming increasingly conscious of the character of each breath. Just as no two snowflakes are exactly the same, the same can be said about each of your breaths. Focus on making your breaths slow, steady and even. Take your time. There is no rush whatsoever and the more relaxed your breath is, the more relaxed your body will be. Breathe as naturally as possible, making the transition from one nostril to the other as smoothly as possible. If you are trying this breathing practice for the first time, spend two to five minutes practicing with your dominant hand and then switch to your non-dominant hand and continue the practice for an additional two to five minutes.

The goal is to nurture and calm yourself with your breath, almost like a gentle internal massage. Be sure to continually refocus your attention on the flow of your breath, releasing any thoughts that float into your mind as you do so. Just put the thoughts on a white fluffy cloud and allow them to drift away as they arise. At first they may come up constantly. Don't let that discourage you. Just continually return your thoughts to your breath.

The reason you will feel so good after engaging in this practice is because this breathing pattern balances the right and left hemispheres of your brain, which creates a strong sense of well-being physically and emotionally. Allow yourself to tune into how your body feels as you oxygenate it, feeding it the healthy nourishment of deep breathing.

Practice #3: Self-Coaching Conversations

A "Self-Coaching Conversation" is an internalized or spoken (out loud) conversation with *yourself* in which you inspire, nurture and guide yourself, in love and compassion, to be with the difficult feelings and to breathe through the urge to binge. In a self-coaching conversation, you will address yourself from the most compassionate, wise and loving part of who you are. Those who feel embarrassed, I invite you to entertain the following question: What do you think is more ridiculous—repeatedly stuffing your feelings down with food and beating yourself up for it afterwards or having a conversation with the part of yourself that is upset? Enough said! Be loving with you!

If you are feeling sad or hurt, ask your inner child what she wants. Keep prodding and asking until you get an answer. Is it a hug? Attention? Does she want you to slow down and spend time doing something fun with her? Is she looking for compassion? A non-food treat of some sort? Often simply by hearing her desires you will find your need for food fades and evaporates. If she is frightened, ask her what she is frightened of. Ask her, "What is the worst thing that could happen here if you don't eat?" When you realize that the overwhelming majority of your fears are phantoms that can be unmasked as soon as you turn the light of your awareness on them, you will relax and trust your life process far more.

A Self-Coaching Conversation is an *extraordinarily* powerful method for bringing yourself into the present moment and from that place making the best possible choices for your body.

I self-coach myself frequently in this way, and it is like having a friendly conversation with someone who cares about me deeply. You can dialogue with yourself frequently throughout the day, any time you find yourself feeling tense, worried or frightened. Just pretend you are talking to a sweet, innocent child if you need a little jump-start to your sweet talk. I found when I talk to myself *out loud*, I am more likely to pay attention to the conversation. I can hear myself with greater clarity. It feels more real to me and is more effective than an internal dialogue. It is one of my self-loving practices that I have found *pivotal* in my ability to move beyond a binge.

Tool #4: Singing Your Song

Music is a profoundly healing tool simply because it has the ability to change your state of mind, drop you into your heart and release you from the endless chatter of the untamed mind. Having a specific song that inspires you can be an extremely effective tool to support you in overcoming a binge. When you feel a powerful urge coming on, sing or hum that song to yourself, either out loud or in your head. The act of singing or humming will support you in creating a state of calm within your body that will again allow you to make a choice from a position of strength rather than one of tension or emotional upset. When you sing, you have to breathe more deeply, which is part of the reason it is so relaxing! Singing is another act of self-love, and a particularly joyous one at that!

Tool #5: Do Something Kind for Someone Else

You can take a significant bite out of an urge to binge by doing something kind for another person. Giving can take your mind off your own discomfort and distract you until you move past a compulsive urge. It can be a simple form of giving, such as taking a moment to send good wishes, pray for, or call someone who you know is going through a hard time. You could make a contribution to a homeless person or find something you are not using and donate it to charity. Sharing builds self-esteem. When you know you have the ability to impact another human being's life in a positive way, you will have an inner feeling of fullness that will temper the urge to eat compulsively. A 1998 survey of overall life satisfaction found that altruistic activity can increase general happiness by twenty-four percent. That's a big dose of happiness as far as I'm concerned! Contributing to someone else's happiness is gourmet food for the soul, an internal feast of fulfillment. Feel free to have a double helping of that!

Tool #6: Do Something Kind for Yourself

If you are reaching for food and you are not physically hungry, you are looking to feel better, calmer or happier. Take a moment to do something kind or loving for yourself and a sense of peace will permeate your body. Write a list of things that feel nurturing to you in the lines provided below. It might be a walk in nature, a hot bath, reading an engrossing novel, a treat like a bottle of pretty nail polish, playing some inspiring music, calling a friend or working on a creative project you've been dreaming about starting. Sometimes temporarily distracting your inner child from thoughts about excess food is helpful to getting beyond the more intense part of the binge urge until the point where you feel capable of withstanding it. Like a child who gets diverted from their momentary obsession through a more appealing distraction, find a way to outsmart your untamed mind by doing something you enjoy!

Tool #7: Get Moving!

If you are feeling anxious, chances are that shallow breathing is contributing to your anxiety. An incredibly helpful way to shift your breathing is by moving your body vigorously. Put on a great song and dance about wildly, take a brisk walk, go for a run, exercise in any way that feels good to your body, scream out loud, do anything different that will shift a shallow breathing pattern to a deep one. Changing your physiology can quell the stress that is at the root of many an urge to binge eat. Exercise that is repetitive in nature (like walking or biking) can give you a meditative, "in the zone" feeling that will calm you as it simultaneously compels you to breathe deeply.

Tool #8: Drink a Glass of Water

As we have previously discussed, drinking a full glass of water will help you to determine if in fact you are thirsty rather than hungry. This simple act can be the equivalent of a splash of cold water against your face, waking you up and out of the old habit of eating compulsively. It's a VERY powerful wake up tool.

Tool #9: Write in Your Journal

Journaling is an opportunity to have a conversation with yourself or your inner child and access the part of yourself that is in fear or stressed. So sit down with your journal and write down your feelings when you have the urge to binge. Next, write down the feeling you would like to have: I want to feel relaxed; I want to feel safe; I want to feel good enough. Sometimes the urge to binge can be completely dissipated through this simple writing process.

Writing after a binge can also contribute to healing your relationship with food. Putting pen to paper and writing about the feelings that you were avoiding can help you to prevent a future binge. When you successfully move beyond the urge to binge, write about it in your journal and dog-ear the journal page that accompanied this victory. This journal entry would be a powerful one to read the next time you are considering eating when you are not hungry. Re-reading it will remind you of how empowering it feels to work out the fears or anxieties driving your emotional appetites.

Tool #10: Turn on Some Inspirational and Soothing Music

Coping with difficult feelings can be challenging, and music is one of life's greatest tools to reduce stress and access peace. According to one study, listening to thirty minutes of calming classical music has the same effect as a ten-milligram dose of Valium! So turn to music instead of marshmallows to give yourself a calm and inspired feeling.

Tool #11: Read an Inspirational Book

Sometimes when I am in an uncomfortable place, all I need to do is to pick up the right book that reminds me of the truth: Life is a glorious journey. Make sure to always have an inspirational book close by to get you to remember how powerful, capable and wonderful you are, or one that reminds you of the indomitable nature of your human spirit.

Tool #12: Professional or Self-Massage

Prior to a binge we unconsciously leave our bodies. We zone out or go on autopilot, ignoring our bodies' communications completely. By massaging our bodies with focus and care, we re-ground and draw ourselves back into our bodies and from that powerful place we can differentiate more easily between our emotional and physical hungers. Remind yourself as you rub your toes how appreciative you are of their role in helping you walk down the street or dance. Rub your arms and send them love for their part in allowing you to embrace those you love.

You will be *far* more likely to make optimum choices when you are in your body, and self-massage can take you there.

If you can afford to receive a professional massage, I recommend doing it as frequently as possible. Nurturing your body in this way is incredibly healing and pleasurable. Additionally, when you recognize the amazing ability of your body to provide you with pleasure, your desire to take care of it will be considerably heightened. Getting a massage sends a message to your body that you value it and want to take excellent care of it. If you have been hard on your body for many years, it most certainly deserves this act of love – and so do you.

Tool #13: Visualization

Visualizing, or imagining, in great detail how you will look and, even more importantly, how you will *feel* at your natural weight is an incredible empowerment tool. Since your subconscious mind does not recognize the difference between what you visualize and what you actually experience in the external world, running the movie of your life at your ideal weight will act as a magnet to create that condition. In one of my all-time favorite movies, "*What the Bleep Do We Know*," the quantum physics' answer to why our thoughts actually *do* create our reality is explained in great detail (it sounds a little dry, but it is absolutely fascinating). If you direct your thoughts towards creating a movie in your mind through visualizing what you want, these thoughts will take you closer to moving the experience from your mind into your physical reality.

Try this visualization. In as much detail as possible, imagine that you around your favorite foods and you are totally comfortable with it. Imagine checking in with your body and realizing you are not hungry; you are happily turning away from the feast for now, knowing that you can return as soon as you are at a Stage Zero/One. Picture yourself smiling and walking away. Imagine yourself turning down an offer for your favorite meal because you are not hungry. Go for the Academy Award of visualizations! Allow the feelings that would accompany the ability to say "Not right now" to any and all food to surge through your body. Feel the sense of strength, power and peace you would experience knowing you can choose not to eat if you are not hungry. The more you allow yourself to visualize and feel the experience, the faster you can manifest the movie in your physical reality. If you can dream it, you can manifest it. This is a fact. If you picture yourself walking away from excess food with a smile on your face every day in your mind's eye, it will make it far easier to do it in your body!

Tool #14: Write Down Ten Things You Are Grateful For

One of the most powerful and life-transforming practices we have at our disposal is gratitude. The opportunity to see and focus on what you *do* have, rather than what you do *not* have, is transformational in terms of your ability to squeeze all of the juice out of life each and every day. Your primitive, fear-driven untamed mind, if not kept in check, would keep you in a continuous state of lack and anxiety. It can be effectively trained away from depleting thoughts through gratitude, and the more the better! Your ability to focus predominantly on the things about your life that you love will allow you to center yourself back in the present moment. I once heard someone say, "It's called the present because it's a gift," and there is tremendous truth in that statement! The present moment is where life unfolds and, if you can focus you attention on being in the now, your life will be a far more enjoyable experience. So back to gratitude. Whenever you feel the urge to binge, take a few moments and write in your journal as many things as you can think of that you are grateful for. Take a moment to revel in your gifts and take comfort in what you have been blessed with. You can transport yourself mentally anywhere from a blush of delight to tears of joy if you *really* think about the things you are most grateful for in your life. You might not get to a place of complete euphoria at first, but at the very least it can take you to a neutral state, which will calm your physiology and allow you to transcend the urge to binge.

Tool #15: For the Good of the Planet

It is an inarguable fact that when you make healthy, loving choices for yourself consistently, you will be a much happier person. And happy people tend to be loving and kind to those around them. In other words, healthy, positive choices for *you* mean a healthier, happier world for others. That's why one of my practices when I feel like I want to eat and I am not hungry, is to encourage myself to wait until I am truly hungry "for the good of the planet." I use my commitment to the betterment of the world as an incentive to feel my uncomfortable feelings and wait until I am legitimately hungry to put any food into my mouth. I don't see it as a sacrifice as much as I do a contribution to something that really matters to me. I know that if I as an individual am able to brave my feelings and withhold harsh self-criticisms, it will add something positive to this planet. I am committed to not allowing my uglier and self-defeating thoughts to pollute a world that I love so much. Consider working through a binge as an act of altruism. It is your gift to the Universe today to choose to wait to eat until you are hungry. By the same token, your gift to the Universe is *also* to be gentle with yourself if you are *unable* to overcome the urge to eat when you were not physically hungry. You don't do anything good, for yourself or the planet, by being mean to yourself.

Tool #16: Spend Quality Time with Your Inner Child

I have a photograph of myself as a newborn baby framed in my bedroom and I look at it daily to remind myself of my true essence, which is innocent and loveable. Oftentimes it is easier for me to look upon myself with compassion if I see myself as that tiny spirit rather than a full-grown adult. Seeing that part of yourself that is an innocent child will support you in softening your heart as you navigate the oftentimes challenging life process.

Put a photo of yourself as a child someplace obvious where you can see it frequently. Allow yourself to feel the tenderness towards yourself that you would feel towards an innocent child. When you are tempted to eat and are not hungry, take that photo of yourself as a child and stare into your own little eyes. Send yourself, both as a child and as an adult, love and compassion for the discomfort you are experiencing. It is your responsibility and glorious opportunity to offer yourself unconditional love. Listen for any requests your inner child might be communicating, and respond to them at your earliest opportunity. This is your chance to re-parent yourself, to give yourself the things you wanted as a child– affection, appreciation, acknowledgement, attention and even outright adoration.

Tool #17: Think of Yourself as "With Child"

There were times in my healing process where I wasn't particularly concerned with what or how I ate. In order to access a gentle place with myself, in order to quiet my untamed mind, which was a barrier to being gentle with myself, I used to think of myself as "with child" (i.e., pregnant). I considered what the impact would be on a little tiny being in my body if I ate unconsciously. Would I be making that little innocent baby sick? Would I be impacting its emotional or physical health negatively? Using that criteria would sometimes stop me dead in my tracks from going into full binge mode. I would make the most loving choices available for my body if I had a child inside of me, out of concern for its well-being. I have learned to use those same loving criteria for my choices for my own health and well-being. With time and practice I was able to offer myself and my body the same level of respect and thoughtfulness.

Tool #18: Call a Friend

Calling a friend, or your co-coach, is a wonderful and highly effective option when faced with a binge urge specifically because they can support you in relaxing, expressing yourself and breathing through the difficult feelings as you get to the root of what is at the core of the urge to binge. Once you find out what is at the root of your urges, you will be able to make a conscious choice to eat or not to eat. Your friend can also encourage you to hold out, feel your emotions and work through them, and help you wait until you are physically hungry by psyching you up to recognize that you are capable of surmounting anything! Often the feeling we are looking for in the form of food can be re-created through a loving conversation with a friend. Studies show that women release a feel-good chemical called "oxytocin" when we talk to each other that improves our overall sense of well-being. By calling a friend, you can receive the same feeling of comfort that you are looking for in food without any of the costs of eating beyond your physical hunger.

*****

The smartest thing you could possibly do if you want to achieve your natural weight is to listen to and honor your body and develop a safe space within yourself to turn to for comfort, guidance, patience and love.

- Lily

Chapter 9

Final Offerings

It took me a very long time to figure out that each and every minute of life is a precious gift. So why would I, or you, want to waste any one of them being hard on ourselves or our bodies? If you want your life to become a more joyous experience, choose instead to spend each moment loving and appreciating yourself, and taking action to transform the circumstances of your life that are not working for you. If you take this wise path, your life will not only match your fondest expectations, it will instead surpass your greatest dreams.

Although everything I have shared in this book can support your goal of creating a healthy relationship with your body and food, the ones I have found to be the most instantly life-transforming are the following six, and I would encourage you to pay special attention to them when you begin the program:

1. Enjoy your meals and give them your undivided attention.

2. Get your body moving through enjoyable forms of exercise regularly.

3. Observe your thoughts and replace negative ones with inspiring and loving ones.

4. Appreciate yourself and be very gentle with yourself when you slip up.

5. Breathe deeply and slow down in your daily life.

6. Regularly remind yourself of all the good things about yourself and your life, be grateful!

7. Talk OUT LOUD to yourself when your untamed mind is suggesting you reach for food when you are not hungry

If you regularly engage in these seven self-love practices, you will both release excess weight and positively impact every aspect of your life. The more you practice these self-loving behaviors, the easier it gets and the more you wake up to your own inherent value.

So here are my final thoughts, a set of inspirations that have helped me to move beyond my eating compulsion and create a life of phenomenal fulfillment.

1. Have more fun.

Being a fun junkie and having more fun now than ever before in my life, I could *easily* write an entire book about the benefits of creating more fun in your life. I'm talking about the kind of pure unadulterated fun where you laugh so hard that tears leak from your eyes and your stomach aches. Where you are having such a great time that you want the day or night to last forever. I'm talking about the magic kind of fun that comes when you are doing *things* you love with *people* you love. Fun is a *mandatory* component for a balanced and whole life experience. If you're not having much fun, something is off and something's gotta give. Fun escapades are the times when your inner child gets to show up and express her playful, carefree, exuberant, adventurous and silly side. If you are not making time for that magical part of who you are, you're going to be cranky, and life is going to feel a little bland. There's no way around it.

Here's what I do and what I invite you to do: Connect with your very best friends, the people you enjoy being with the most and let them know you want to have more fun in your life and you want to include them in it. (Who's gonna say no to that?!) Then brainstorm about things you can do together that have an inherently high fun factor. Be imaginative and unrestrained. Put some time into defining your ideas; write them on a list and introduce more of them back into your life one by one. Be spontaneous. Whether it's climbing into a jumpy house with your kids at a birthday party, getting gussied up for a night of dancing, taking a bike ride by the beach, planning a girls weekend, going to live music concerts or getting dressed up for Halloween, step outside your normal routine. If you just started a co-coaching relationship, encourage each other to have more fun and share as many fun activities with each other as humanly possible given your respective schedules.

Don't hold back. Make the fun factor your priority. Make time for it every day, even if it is for ten minutes. A healthy balance between work, play and leisure time will suffuse the emotional hungers that were present because you weren't living the "fun-tastic" (corny, but accurate) life you needed and wanted. The more fun you are having, the more full you will feel! Having a good time reduces the compulsive eating urges because instead of looking for different flavors solely through food, you will find them in your life!

2. Slow down.

I used to live life on the fast track, where my schedule was so full that I could rarely take a break and not feel guilty or worry that I was going to fall way behind. There were *many* times I wanted to step off that fast track but didn't know how. I simply had too much to do. I prioritized my life in a way that didn't allow for *nearly* as much relaxation and fun as I wanted or, as it turns out, needed. Because my schedule was imbalanced and overly busy, my untamed mind thoughts were on overdrive. From experience I know that without balance in your life, the untamed mind will get much louder and stronger and will continue to feed an "I can't do anything about it" attitude. Now, at the glorious age of forty-four, I balance my life between the slow lane and the fast lane. I still love the productivity that comes with jammin' on my to do list, but I also create lots and lots of downtime where I do things I find rejuvenating, creative and inspiring. I have had to make some lifestyle changes to accommodate this new way of being, but I don't think I even need to tell you how worthwhile it was! If you want to progress faster in your life in terms of your personal happiness, give the *slow* a go. Practice by eating slower, driving slower, making decisions slower and making space amid all the doing and just *be*. Hang out in your garden and breathe or take a stroll in a beautiful park. Mother Nature is the best place I can think of to just be. These slow times are the ones where it is much easier to connect with the voice of sweetness within you because your tamed mind is not so preoccupied with tasks and responsibilities. Going slowly also reduces the hasty eating that goes hand in hand with being overly busy and keeps me grounded in my body and centered in the present moment. You don't have to grind your life to a screeching halt, just ease up gradually. The first step is to slow down long enough to determine your priorities and then to develop a game plan for living in sync with them.

3. **Let go of perfectionism.**

I am not perfect, nor do I plan on shooting for my untamed mind's crazy, exhausting, insatiable and unrealistic image of perfection ever again. Perfection is a subjectively chosen illusion that will drive *anyone* living on planet Earth crazy. You will run yourself ragged trying to live up to your own idea of perfection. In contrast to the past, today I love owning my *imperfection*. I feel like I've broken free from an evil stepmother who kept me busy working so that I didn't have time to have, or get to, the ball, where everyone else was having a great time. I see myself, and all human beings for that matter, as "perfectly imperfect." Sure I have areas of my life where I can admit that my low-vibration behaviors are still a little more present than I would like. But instead of being ashamed of my shadow qualities and denying them in myself because I found them so unappealing, I now allow myself to acknowledge those parts of who I am; I have learned to be forgiving and gentle with myself. I know that all of my low-vibration behaviors in their extreme are a result of fear: fear of not being enough or having enough. I have finally created a safe space within myself where I can admit to my shadow traits, which frees me up to move beyond them with greater grace and ease. When I had no safe space, I couldn't admit to them because I would make myself feel horrible and beat myself up for my mistakes and imperfections. Whereas being hard and unforgiving of myself made me a more judgmental, fearful and intolerant person, loving myself has bought out the best of who I am, my kinder, more loving, compassionate side. Simply stated, self-love made me a much better person. I believe that when every one of us loves ourselves even a *little* bit more, it will bring about massive positive change not only in our personal lives, but also in the world at large. A little self-love goes a *looooong* way.

If perfectionism is a theme in your life that you'd love to shift, make it your goal to cut yourself as many breaks as possible so that you can bring the best of who *you* are to the table and be an active participant in making this world a better place. You have my passionate support in that noble intention!

4. Enjoy the processes in your life.

I have finally embraced the perspective that *what* I get accomplished during the day is not *nearly* as important as *who I am being* as I'm getting it done. Almost everything I can think of in life involves a process—whether it's writing a book, getting kids off to school or getting dressed in the morning. A *series* of processes are what every day is made of. It *finally* dawned on me that if I am only satisfied when the "it" I am dealing with is over and done with, instead of enjoying the process, I'd have very few joyous moments. I'll spend the overwhelming majority of my life in a state of angst and dissatisfaction waiting impatiently for the finished moments.

Not being able to relax as I went about my day was part of the reason I ate compulsively. I ate nervously instead of luxuriously. I have learned not to measure the quality of my days based exclusively upon my accomplishments, but rather by the joy I experienced. If I have a super-productive day and am cranky, it doesn't feel nearly as good as having a balanced day where I enjoy every morsel of it (or many more of them at the very least). The days where I put my energy into *being in the moment* are *much* more fulfilling and make me happier to be alive—and from what others tell me, easier to be around.

5. Believe in yourself.

If you *really* want to expedite your healing process, *believe in yourself.* Although others can support you with this goal, no one can do it for you.

It is your soul journey and your responsibility. You have got to be the one who has more faith in you than anyone else, who loves you more than anyone else. You get to be your mentor, unwavering supporter, loudest cheerleader and safe space. Make it your daily intention to raise the bar on your thoughts, *especially* the thoughts you entertain about yourself.

Slow down and listen for that sweet voice in your head, the one that is gentle and understanding, the one that offers you the most loving and high-vibration perspective you can think of. Heed its messages. They are pearls of wisdom that will guide you to your soul's destination–to be a living model of love, love of yourself and consequently love of others. There is only one of you in this world and you are as *precious* as any member of this planet. You have been given an opportunity through the challenges you face with food to tap into the depths of your being, and when you do so, your own magnificence will be revealed to you. Prepare to fall deeply in love with yourself!

6. Practice Gratitude.

Every religion in the world incorporates the practice of gratitude, so you *know* there's something special about this act! Although I touched upon this topic in various spots throughout this book, I felt it deserved one more mention given its extraordinary power. In my past, my focus on my body and what I didn't like about it garnered a huge amount of my attention. It was difficult for me to appreciate *anything* given that my focus was almost always on what I didn't have in terms of my body. No wonder I felt depressed! And I didn't learn until much later in life that gratitude is an incredibly powerful anti-depressant! Every day of my life I actively search for the things I am grateful for, whether it's a good parking space or a sweet comment from one of the wonderful children in my life. My appreciation for the little things and the big things has been a powerful mood-enhancing tool that allows me to find massive satisfaction in every day. It is miraculous. As an added bonus, the more I focus on what I have to be grateful for, the more I attract things to be grateful for. This simple practice of appreciation draws in a gold mine of riches, both spiritual and financial. If you want to open the floodgates of abundance, give thanks!

Parting Words

So those are my final insights and invitations to you, dear reader, and I am grateful to have had the opportunity to share them. It has been a deeply healing experience for me to write this book and give to others the information and perspectives I had wished for in my most desperate moments. Looking back on the tougher parts of my history, I know I am a far stronger, kinder, compassionate, understanding and loving person having experienced compulsions with food and body disconnection. Although I would not want to repeat the experience of being obsessed with food, it has been a great teacher in my life, one for which I am (I can't believe I'm writing this) grateful for in retrospect (but only in retrospect). Huge personal growth came to me in the darkest times of my life, through my emotional discomfort and my willingness to stop avoiding it and face it square in the eye. By doing so I increased my fearlessness, my self-respect, my awareness of my power, my willpower and my joy.

If you look carefully at your own life, you too will see that your issues around food and your body have provided you with the motivation to deeply contemplate yourself and your life. Through intense misery and desperation in many cases, you were forced to ask yourself the deeper questions that allowed you to know yourself on a more intimate level and think about life on a much broader level. If you are willing to embrace the lessons that the tough times have offered your soul's development, your compulsion around food, having served its purpose, can be more easily released.

After years of low self-esteem and self-denigration, I have come to a place where today, I can say without hesitation that I love myself. My daily goal is to love myself with the tender and endless love that a mother has for her child. Because I choose this "road less traveled," repeatedly my life is a reflection of more peace, fun, joy and celebration than I ever dreamed possible.

Remember, you offer a light to this world that *no one* else can and it shines most brightly when you offer yourself love and respect. It is time to claim your birthright of self-love and start enjoying the extravagantly exquisite gift of life on higher levels. I wish you *every* happiness you can fathom on your life journey. Love and peace galore, Lily

###

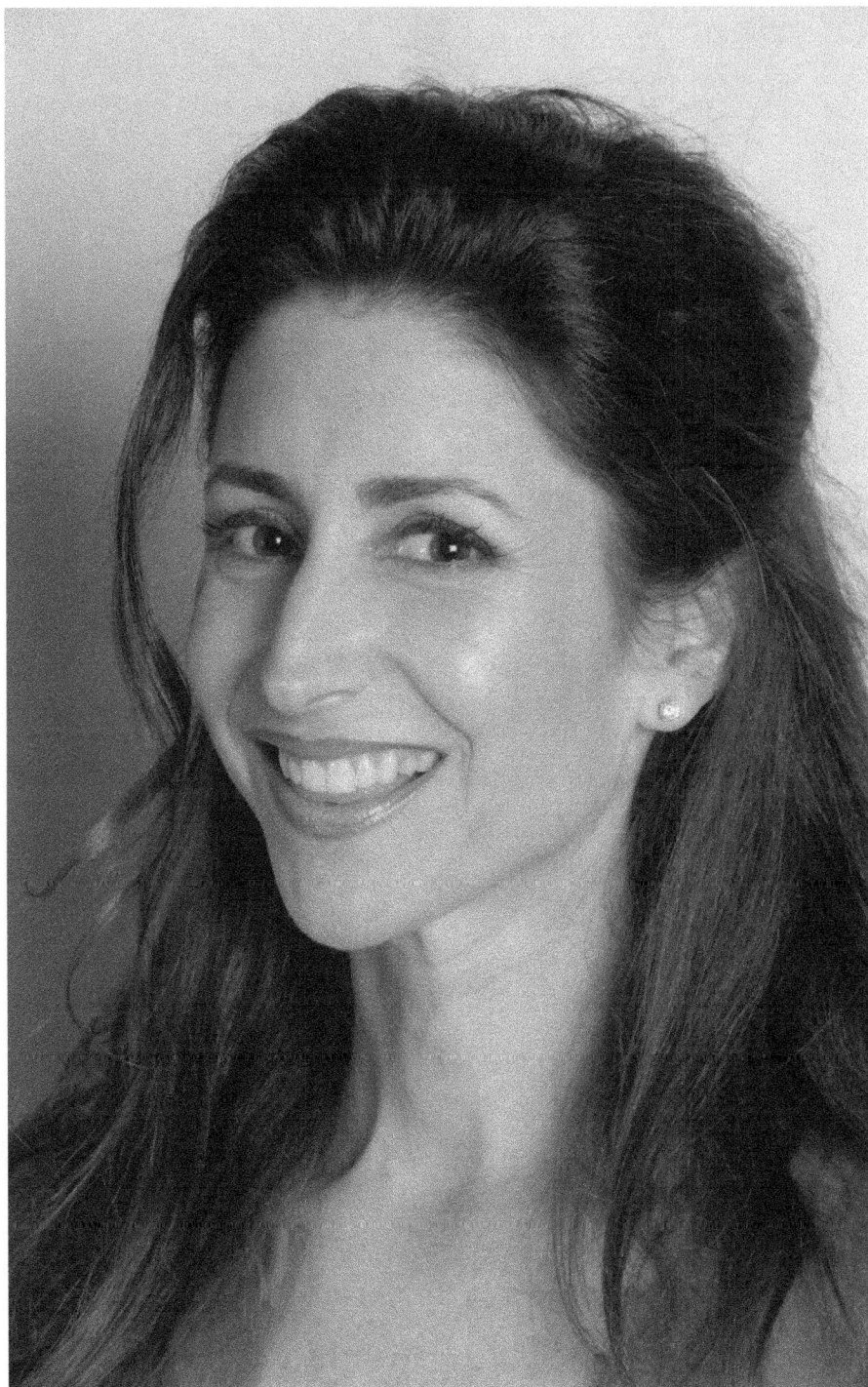

About the Author

Elizabeth "Lily" Hills is a multiple award winning author, international inspirational/motivational public speaker, and corporate trainer. She is the former radio host for sparkpeople.com, the #1 online health site in America with over 16 million members. Her recent passion project is The Mindful Eating Method, the most comprehensive online training in the world for overcoming overeating. She created it for those who were ready to give up dieting and wanted to have 24/7 support as they moved away from emotional eating habits. Her purpose is supporting others in learning the life transforming practice of self-love. She currently lives (gratefully) in Carmel, California.

Connect With Lily

http://www.TheMindfulEatingMethod.com/

Appendix B:

Here are two associations that keep a register of professionals who specialize in helping those with eating disorder issues. To find support in your area please contact one of the following organizations:

National Association of Anorexia Nervosa and Associated Disorders (ANAD)

P.O. Box 7

Highland Park, IL 60035

Phone: 1-847-831-3438

Website: ANAD.org

E-mail: ANADhelp@ANAD.org

All ANAD services are offered free to the public

National Eating Disorders Association (NEDA)

603 Stewart Street, Suite 803

Seattle, WA 98101

Phone: 1-206-382-3587

Website: NationalEatingDisorders.org

Email: info@NationalEatingDisorders.org

Toll-free Information and Referral Helpline: 1-800-931-2237

Helpline hours are 8:30 a.m. to 4:30 p.m. Pacific Time.

All NEDA services are offered free to the public

www.ingramcontent.com/pod-product-compliance
Lightning Source LLC
Chambersburg PA
CBHW021501090426
42739CB00007B/413